Test Bank for

Essentials of
Maternal-Newborn
Nursing

Test Bank for

Essentials of
Maternal-Newborn
Nursing
Second Edition

PATRICIA WIELAND LADEWIG

MARCIA L. LONDON

SALLY BROOKENS OLDS

ADDISON-WESLEY NURSING
A Division of The Benjamin/Cummings Publishing Company, Inc.

Redwood City, California • Fort Collins, Colorado • Menlo Park, California
Reading, Massachusetts • New York • Don Mills, Ontario • Wokingham, U.K.
Amsterdam • Bonn • Sydney • Singapore • Tokyo • Madrid • San Juan

Sponsoring Editor: Doug Thornburg
Cover Designer: Detta Penna

ISBN 0-201-53238-7

ABCDEFGHIJ--MU--8932109

ADDISON-WESLEY NURSING
A Division of The Benjamin/Cummings Publishing Company, Inc.
390 Bridge Parkway
Redwood City, California 94065

PREFACE

This Test Bank to accompany the second edition of <u>Essentials of Maternal-Newborn Nursing</u> by Patricia Ladewig, Marcia London, and Sally Olds has been revised for the new edition of their bestselling text. In this Test Bank you will find almost 800 multiple-choice questions, including test items for new content on Maternal Nutrition, Newborn Nutrition, Women's Health Care, and The Childbearing Family: Age-Related Considerations. Test questions now have greater emphasis on application and comprehension of concepts, rather than straight recall of information. This gives you the opportunity to test students the way you'd prefer: with applications to real-world nursing situations that reinforce critical thinking.

The Test Bank offers thorough and comprehensive coverage of the text material and provides an easy-to-use database from which you can create numerous unique examinations quickly and efficiently. The Test Bank is offered to adopters of the text in two forms for maximum flexibility: the printed Test Bank manual, or a microcomputer disk for the IBM PC or Apple Macintosh computer, to be used with the Delta testing software. This software allows you to scramble the order in which questions appear on the exams you create, as well as to scramble the multiple-choice options within a question. You can also choose questions based on the classification system described below. You can choose your own combination of questions, and you can add up to an additional 300 questions of your design. If you have questions about the Delta computerized test-generating program, please contact your Addison-Wesley sales representative at 1-800-950-5544.

For your convenience, the test items have been classified in the left margin of your manual in the following manner:

NUMBERING: The test items are modeled on the NCLEX standard: real-life nursing situations (scenarios) with several related multiple-choice questions referring to each scenario. The questions are numbered by chapter and item number (1-1, 1-2, and so on).

ANSWER: The correct answer to each questions appears underneath the test item number.

NURSING PROCESS STEP: Each question is classified according to nursing process, as follows:

Asses.	=	Assessment
Analy.	=	Analysis/Diagnosis
Plan.	=	Planning
Impl.	=	Implementation
Eval.	=	Evaluation

COGNITIVE LEVEL: A cognitive level has been selected that is appropriate for the item, as follows:

Know.	=	Knowledge
Comp.	=	Comprehension
Appl.	=	Application

This Test Bank manual was developed with you, the instructor, in mind. The authors, editors, and publisher have sought to provide you with a testing package that offers quality test items, flexibility, variety, and accuracy. We hope you find it useful.

ACKNOWLEDGEMENTS

The authors would like to thank the nurses who provided test questions to accompany the third edition of <u>Maternal-Newborn Nursing: A Family-Centered Approach.</u> Many of their questions have been used or adapted for this book. They are: Marsha Irwin, RN, MEd, MED-ED Associates, North Harris County College; Jeanne Lowell, MSN, RNC, Central Oklahoma Community Mental Health Center; Berthine Mason, RN, MN, North Harris County College; Gail Maxwell, RN, MS, University of Oklahoma; Fay McClay, RN, PhD, North Harris County College; Judy Walker, RN, EdD, North Harris County College; Francene Weatherby, RNC, MSN, MA, University of Oklahoma; and Virginia Zizelmann, RN, PhD, North Harris County College.

CONTENTS

PART I

BASIC CONCEPTS

Chapter 1

Contemporary Maternal-Newborn Care

Instructions: For each of the following multiple-choice questions, select the ONE most appropriate answer.

1-1
B
Comp.
N/A

As a nurse gains more experience, s/he is able to:

a. prevent complications associated with childbirth.
b. view clinical situations in a holistic manner.
c. move into teaching positions.
d. manage complex clinical situations without supervision.

1-2
A
Comp.
N/A

Contemporary childbirth focuses on:

a. family-centered care.
b. free-standing birthing centers.
c. outpatient childbirth.
d. strict infection control measures.

1-3
C
Comp.
Diag.

Which of the following statements is TRUE concerning early discharge following childbirth?

a. Neonates often return to the hospital with respiratory infections.
b. Nurses do not include adequate teaching in their discharge planning.
c. Many clients are not emotionally ready to learn neonatal and self-care.
d. Early discharge often results in postpartum hemorrhage.

1-4
B
Comp.
Analy.

Nurses are moving in the direction of using the term "client" rather than "patient" because:

a. insurance companies are more likely to provide compensation when the term "client" is used.
b. the term "client" implies an active role in health care.
c. the term "client" implies a degree of detachment on the part of the nurse.
d. the term "client" sounds better than "patient."

1-5
C
Comp.
Analy.

The cornerstone of health teaching for the childbearing woman is:

a. formalized teaching in a group setting.
b. focusing on physiological changes associated with pregnancy.
c. individualized teaching at the woman's level of understanding.
d. inclusion of all family members in the teaching process.

1-6 Many physicians have abandoned obstetric care because:
D
Comp. a. there is less interest in obstetrics/gynecology.
Analy. b. fewer women are becoming pregnant.
  c. there are more home births than in the past.
  d. insurance premiums have significantly escalated.

1-7 A PRIMARY crisis faced by certified nurse midwives is:
A
Comp. a. escalation of malpractice insurance rates.
Analy. b. lack of trust by the health care consumer.
  c. not enough childbearing business.
  d. inadequate obstetrical facilities.

1-8 A minimum standard of care, required of all professional nurses, refers to:
B
Comp. a. the least amount of nursing care for safe practice.
Analy. b. the care that a reasonable, prudent nurse would provide in a particular situation.
  c. nursing care as described in policy manuals.
  d. staffing patterns which prescribe a minimum number of professional nurses to
    provide good care.

1-9 The individual responsible for obtaining an informed consent from the client is the:
C
Know. a. admissions officer.
Analy. b. nurse.
  c. physician.
  d. unit secretary.

1-10 The only legal evidence that can substantiate that a nurse has made adequate client
D assessments, provided quality care, and notified the physician when necessary is:
Know.
Analy. a. the audiotape from the change-of-shift report.
  b. testimony under oath in a court of law.
  c. statements from co-workers who observed the nurse's actions.
  d. documentation in the client's chart.

1-11 Laura Stanley, RN, was the circulating nurse during a cesarean birth. It was later
C discovered that a sponge was left in the incision, and the client developed a severe
Know. infection requiring further surgery. Which of the following statements is TRUE
Analy. concerning legal aspects of the situation?

  a. It is the physician's responsibility to provide adequate care in the management of
    surgical wounds.
  b. There is minimal legal risk because the nurse acted in good faith.
  c. The nurse could be cited for clinical negligence by failing to accurately account for
    all sponges.
  d. The hospital would be held primarily responsible and would be covered by its
    malpractice insurance.

2

1-12
D
Know.
Analy.

Effective risk management in maternal-child care should focus on:

a. evaluation of incidents by a legal issues committee.
b. creating a totally safe environment for client care.
c. skills training workshops for all maternal-child staff.
d. taking prompt action to prevent incidents from occurring.

1-13
A
Appl.
Impl.

Cathy and John Fullerton are considering surrogate childbearing, but Cathy is concerned about her legal status as the child's mother. Which of the following replies would be the most appropriate nursing response?

a. "The biological mother will retain legal custody."
b. "That is not an issue as long as you all agree to the process."
c. "Cathy, you will legally adopt the child."
d. "That is just one of many problems you will face if you decide to go through with this."

1-14
D
Know.
Analy.

Legal issues associated with in vitro fertilization (IVF) and embryo transfer (ET) include questions about:

a. what to do with embryos that are not implanted.
b. what to do when a multiple pregnancy occurs.
c. paternity if donor sperm are used.
d. all of these.

1-15
B
Know.
N/A

Certified nurse-midwives do which of the following:

a. attend home births under the direction of a physician.
b. give primary care to healthy women during pregnancy, birth, and postpartum.
c. give high-risk care for patients if they are in hospital settings.
d. have physicians present for any technical procedures.

1-16
D
Know.
Analy.

The maternal-newborn nurse bases her/his practice on:

a. anatomical and physiological concepts.
b. sociological and culturally acceptable norms.
c. a comprehensive, interdisciplinary knowledge base.
d. all of these.

1-17
C
Know.
Asses.

During the assessment phase of the nursing process, the nurse collects both objective and subjective data. Objective data includes all of the following EXCEPT:

a. laboratory test results.
b. head-to-toe physical examination.
c. the client's perception of the childbearing process.
d. vital signs.

1-18
B
Know.
Diag.

In contrast to the medical diagnosis, the nursing diagnosis:

a. is not included in the woman's medical record.
b. reflects the changing response of the woman to her condition.
c. has little, if any, bearing on care the woman receives.
d. generally remains the same throughout the woman's health problem.

1-19   Outcome goals are established:
C
Comp.   a. when the woman is admitted for obstetric care.
Plan.   b. after specific interventions have been identified.
         c. after the analysis is completed and nursing diagnoses are formulated.
         d. prior to discharge or referral to other agencies.

1-20   During the evaluation phase of the nursing process, the expected outcomes (goals)
A   should be evaluated by the:
Know.
Eval.   a. woman and the nurse.
         b. nurse and the physician.
         c. supervisor of maternal-child nursing.
         d. woman and her physician.

1-21   There are two types of statistics: descriptive and inferential. An example of descriptive
B   statistics is:
Know.
Analy.   a. a positive correlation between two or more variables.
         b. the infant mortality rate in Oklahoma.
         c. a causal relationship between two events.
         d. the total number of spontaneous abortions in drug abusing women.

1-22   The type of statistic that answers specific questions and generates theories to explain
C   phenomena is:
Know.
N/A   a. descriptive.
         b. qualitative.
         c. inferential.
         d. nominal.

1-23   The term "birth rate" refers to:
A
Know.   a. the number of live births per 1000 population.
Analy.   b. the number of live births each year.
         c. the average number of births for a given woman.
         d. the number of births per 1000 women aged 15 to 44 in a given population.

1-24   The low birth weight infant weighs:
B
Know.   a. 3150 g or less.
Analy.   b. less than 2500 g.
         c. less than 3600 g.
         d. 3200 g or less.

1-25   "Neonatal mortality" is defined as the number of deaths of infants less than _____
A   per 1000 live births.
Know.
Analy.   a. 28 days of age
         b. 1 month of age
         c. 15 days of age
         d. 1 week of age

1-26   "Fetal death" refers to:
C
Know.   a. birth of a stillborn neonate.
Analy. b. the total number of spontaneously aborted fetuses.
        c. death in utero at 20 weeks or more gestation.
        d. the number of stillbirths per 1000 live births.

1-27   The four leading causes of infant death include all of the following conditions
D   EXCEPT:
Know.
Analy. a. respiratory distress syndrome.
        b. congenital abnormalities.
        c. sudden infant death syndrome (SIDS).
        d. failure to thrive syndrome secondary to maternal deprivation.

1-28   The maternal death rate in the last 25 years has:
A
Know.   a. steadily decreased.
Analy. b. shown no significant changes over time.
        c. shown consistent increases.
        d. increased because of additional stresses encountered by the woman.

1-29   Factors influencing the decrease in maternal mortality include all of the following
B   EXCEPT:
Know.
Analy. a. the establishment of high risk centers.
        b. use of birth control to prevent pregnancy.
        c. prevention and control of infection.
        d. improved obstetric techniques and anesthesia.

1-30   Maternal-child nurses can make use of applied statistics in all of the following ways
D   EXCEPT:
Know.
Analy. a. in determining populations at risk.
        b. in assessing relationships among variables.
        c. in establishing a data base for a variety of populations.
        d. by directly observing family lifestyle over time.

1-31   In order for nursing research to be successful, it must:
C
Know.   a. be conducted by graduate level practitioners.
Analy. b. focus on large sample sizes.
        c. be useful to nurses in clinical settings.
        d. involve many variables and nursing concepts.

1-32   One of the nurse's initial responsibilities in teaching the pregnant adolescent client is to:
D
Comp.   a. advise her about proper care of the infant.
Impl.   b. instruct her about danger signs of pregnancy-induced hypertension.
        c. instruct her about special concerns of pregnancy.
        d. impress her with the importance of regular attendance at the clinic.

1-33
B
Comp.
Analy.

The use of the nursing process is important in maternal-newborn nursing care because:

a. nursing standards require it for accreditation.
b. it represents a logical approach to problem solving.
c. it keeps charts and knowledge about patients consistent among nurses.
d. it reduces the work load of nurses.

1-34
C
Know.
Asses.

Statistics that describe the number of maternal deaths are called:

a. maternal morbidity rates.
b. maternal illness rates.
c. maternal mortality rates.
d. none of these.

Chapter 2

Reproductive Anatomy and Physiology

Instructions: For each of the following multiple-choice questions, select the ONE most appropriate answer.

Susan Jannis, a senior nursing student, is speaking to a young people's group on the changes that occur during puberty.

(THE FOLLOWING 6 ITEMS RELATE TO THE ABOVE PASSAGE.)

2-1
D
Know
N/A

Susan begins her discussion by defining puberty. The best definition is, "Puberty is the period:

a. when adult sexual characteristics and functions are attained."
b. immediately prior to the development of adult sexual characteristics and functions."
c. of development of adult characteristics more than the development of adult functions."
d. between childhood and the attainment of adult sexual characteristics and functions."

2-2
A
Know.
Asses.

One of the male group members asks Susan how he could tell he was approaching puberty. Her best reply would be, "The physical changes that precede puberty in boys include:

a. the appearance of pubic, axillary, and facial hair; increase in the size of the external genitals; and deepening of the voice."
b. the appearance of pubic, axillary, and facial hair, and nocturnal emissions that contain mature sperm."
c. increase in the size of the external genitals, a higher pitch of the voice, and broadening of the hips."
d. decrease in the rate of growth, facial hair, and broadening of the hips."

2-3
B
Appl.
Asses.

One of the girls in the group asks, "What is the relationship between breast development and the onset of menstruation?" Susan's best reply would be:

a. "Menstruation usually begins about 2 to 3 years before breast development begins."
b. "The average time between breast development and the onset of menstruation is about 2 years."
c. "There is no relationship between breast development and menstruation."
d. "The onset of menstruation is related to the appearance of pubic and axillary hair more than it is to breast development."

2-4
D
Know.
Asses.

Susan explains that puberty is initiated by the maturation of:

a. androgens of estrogens.
b. the anterior pituitary.
c. the hypothalamus.
d. the gonads.

2-5
D
Appl.
Asses.

Another girl in the group asks Susan if the female breasts have any function other than providing nourishment to babies. Susan's best reply is:

a. "No, the only function of the female breast is to breast-feed babies."
b. "The main function of the female breast is to provide pleasurable, sexual sensations."
c. "The main function of the female breast is to nourish and to provide a source of antibodies to babies."
d. "The function of the female breast is to nourish and to provide a source of antibodies to babies. In addition, it serves as a source of sexual sensation."

2-6
C
Appl.
Asses.

Another boy in the group asks if the scrotum serves a function. Susan's best reply is: "The scrotum:

a. serves no function that we know of at this time."
b. is a highly insensitive structure that houses the testicles."
c. protects the testes and the sperm."
d. maintains a higher temperature environment than the body does."

2-7
B
Know.
Asses.

The average age for the onset of puberty in girls is:

a. 9 years of age.
b. 12 years of age.
c. 14 years of age.
d. 17 years of age.

2-8
B
Know.
Asses.

In the female, the gametes are produced by the:

a. vagina.
b. ovaries.
c. uterus.
d. fallopian tubes.

2-9
C
Know.
Asses.

In the male, the gametes are produced by the:

a. penis.
b. prostate.
c. testes.
d. vas deferens.

2-10
B
Know.
Asses.

For fertilization to occur, what portion of the sperm must enter the ovum?

a. the entire sperm.
b. only the head.
c. only the tail.
d. either the head or the tail.

2-11
B
Know.
Asses.

Approximately _____ ova are released during the reproductive years.

a. 200
b. 400
c. 2000
d. 4000

2-12 The perineal body of the female is:
D
Comp.   a. equal in size to the perineal body of the male.
Analy. b. smaller in size than the perineal body of the male.
        c. slightly larger than the perineal body of the male.
        d. much larger than the perineal body of the male.

2-13 During a routine pelvic examination, the clinician can visually examine the:
D
Know.   a. body of the uterus.
Asses. b. fallopian tubes.
        c. ovaries.
        d. uterine cervix.

2-14 The true pelvis is composed of the portions of the pelvis which:
B
Know.   a. lie above the linea terminalis.
N/A   b. lie below the promontory of the sacrum, the linea terminalis, and the upper
           margin of the pubic bones.
        c. lie above the upper border of the linea terminalis and the tuberosities of the ishium.
        d. lie below the ishial spines.

2-15 The function of the Skene's ducts (paraurethral glands) is to:
D
Know.   a. aid micturition.
Asses. b. secrete a spermicidal secretion to aid in birth control.
        c. secrete neutral vaginal secretions to aid in fertilization.
        d. facilitate sexual intercourse by lubricating the vagina.

2-16 The primary components of the external female reproductive system are the:
C
Know.   a. clitoris, vaginal canal, and perineal body.
Asses. b. labia, clitoris, urethra, and perineal body.
        c. mons, labia, and clitoris.
        d. mons, labia, and vagina.

2-17 The layer of the nonpregnant uterus that undergoes monthly regeneration and
C   renewal is the:
Know.
Asses. a. perimetrium.
        b. myometrium.
        c. endometrium.
        d. corpus of the uterus.

2-18 The layer of the uterus most involved with the birth of the fetus is the:
B
Comp.   a. perimetrium.
Asses. b. myometrium.
        c. mucosa.
        d. endometrium.

2-19
C
Comp.
Asses.

A portion of postpartum assessment includes visual inspection of the perineum. The perineum is the area:

a. surrounding the vagina.
b. between the mons pubis and the anus.
c. between the vagina and the anus.
d. between the clitoris and the anus.

2-20
C
Know.
Asses.

The hormone(s) primarily responsible for the development of female secondary sexual characteristics is/are:

a. FSH and LH.
b. GnRF.
c. estrogen and progesterone.
d. ACTH and STH.

2-21
A
Know.
Asses.

The hormone primarily responsible for the development of male secondary sexual characteristics is:

a. testosterone.
b. GnRF.
c. ACTH.
d. thyroid.

2-22
D
Know.
Asses.

The follicle-stimulating hormone (FSH) and luteinizing hormone (LH) are secreted by the:

a. hypothalamus.
b. ovaries and testes.
c. CNS.
d. anterior pituitary.

2-23
A
Know.
Asses.

The bony limits of the birth canal are represented by the:

a. true pelvis.
b. false pelvis.
c. major pelvis.
d. greater pelvis.

2-24
D
Know.
Asses.

The diameter of the female pelvis that determines if the fetus can progress downward into the birth canal is the:

a. conjugate vera.
b. transverse diameter.
c. diagonal conjugate.
d. obstetric conjugate.

2-25
D
Comp.
Asses.

A pregnant adolescent asks the nurse, "How can a woman's body stretch enough for a baby to come out without tearing?" The perineal body is able to stretch without tearing during childbirth because of:

a. a toned and elastic pubococcygeal muscle.
b. hormonal changes associated with pregnancy.
c. increased blood supply.
d. muscles mingled with elastic fibers and connective tissue.

2-26
A
Know.
Asses.

The hormone primarily responsible for the development of female characteristics is:

a. estrogen.
b. progesterone.
c. FSH.
d. LH.

2-27
A
Know.
Asses.

The hormone that increases contractions in the uterus is:

a. estrogen.
b. progesterone.
c. FSH.
d. LH.

2-28
B
Know.
Asses.

Which of the following four phases of the menstrual cycle is eliminated if implantation occurs?

a. menorrhagia phase
b. ischemic phase
c. menarcheal phase
d. menidrosis phase

2-29
B
Comp.
Analy.

The hormone that prepares the uterus for implantation of the fertilized ovum and helps to maintain pregnancy is:

a. estrogen.
b. progesterone.
c. FSH.
d. LH.

2-30
A
Know.
Asses.

The endometrium is shed during which phase of the menstrual cycle?

a. menstrual phase
b. proliferative phase
c. secretory phase
d. ischemic phase

2-31
B
Know.
Asses.

The endometrium thickens during which phase of the menstrual cycle?

a. menstrual phase
b. proliferative phase
c. secretory phase
d. ischemic phase

2-32
C
Know.
Asses.

The vascularity of the uterus increases and the endometrium becomes prepared for a fertilized ovum in which phase of the menstrual cycle?

a. menstrual phase
b. proliferative phase
c. secretory phase
d. ischemic phase

2-33
D
Know.
Asses.

The corpus luteum begins to degenerate, the estrogen and progesterone levels fall, and the blood supply to the endometrium is reduced in which phase of the menstrual cycle?

a. menstrual phase
b. proliferative phase
c. secretory phase
d. ischemic phase

Chapter 3

Women's Health Care

Instructions: For each of the following multiple-choice questions, select the ONE most appropriate answer.

Joanne Parker, RN, is the office nurse for a gynecologist.

(THE FOLLOWING 2 ITEMS RELATE TO THE ABOVE PASSAGE.)

3-1
A
Know.
Asses.

Joanne escorts Mrs. King and her 14-year-old daughter, Karen, to the examination room. As Joanne asks Mrs. King and Karen the reason for their visit, Mrs. King explains that Karen has never had a menstrual period and that she is concerned there may be something wrong. As Joanne writes in Karen's chart, she uses the medical term _____, which indicates the onset of menstruation.

    a. menarche
    b. climacteric
    c. amenorrhea
    d. gynecomastia

3-2
C
Appl.
Diag.

The diagnosis that most correctly describes Karen's condition is:

    a. primary dysmenorrhea.
    b. primary infertility.
    c. primary amenorrhea.
    d. secondary amenorrhea.

3-3
B
Know.
Asses.

Another patient, Bertha Jones, is complaining of having heavier bleeding than normal during her menstrual period. Joanne correctly documents this subjective information in Bertha's chart as:

    a. metrorrhagia.
    b. menorrhagia.
    c. polymenorrhea.
    d. hypermenorrhea.

3-4
C
Appl.
Impl.

Mrs. Jones asks Joanne if it is okay for her to take a tub bath while she is bleeding so heavily. Joanne's best response would be:

    a. "Tub baths are contraindicated during menstruation."
    b. "Tub baths or showers and daily douching are highly recommended."
    c. "Either a bath or shower is fine at this time."
    d. "Bathing, use of a sitz bath, and use of a feminine deodorant spray are all highly recommended during menstruation."

3-5
C
Appl.
Impl.

Mrs. Jones also asks Joanne about the use of tampons while her menstrual flow is heavy. The best advice from Joanne would be:

a. "Tampons should be avoided when the menstrual flow is heavy."
b. "Super tampons with added deodorants are recommended for the day, while regular tampons may be worn at night."
c. "Tampons should only be used during the days when the menstrual flow is heavy; change to napkins at night."
d. "Tampons are recommended for use at the end of the menstrual period rather than at the beginning of the period."

Judy Hoyle, 32 years old, is complaining of frequent headaches, irritability, depression, and breast tenderness associated with her menstrual periods. Her gynecologist diagnoses premenstrual syndrome.

(THE FOLLOWING 5 ITEMS RELATE TO THE ABOVE PASSAGE.)

3-6
D
Appl.
Diag.

The cluster of symptoms Judy presents is the result of a/an:

a. increase in estrogen production.
b. decrease in estrogen production.
c. increase in progesterone production.
d. decrease in progesterone production.

3-7
C
Comp.
Analy.

Judy's age, when compared to that of other women who have premenstrual syndrome, is:

a. lower.
b. higher.
c. characteristic of most women with this condition.
d. not significant.

3-8
A
Appl.
Impl.

The nurse should counsel Judy regarding her diet and should recommend Judy avoid:

a. caffeinated beverages and chocolate cake.
b. high starch foods such as potatoes and spaghetti.
c. fatty foods such as ground beef and pork.
d. breads and cereals.

3-9
A
Appl.
Impl.

Judy asks if vitamins help reduce the symptoms of PMS. The nurse replies that the vitamins which seem to be most helpful are:

a. vitamins B complex and E.
b. vitamins C and E.
c. vitamins A and C.
d. vitamins A and D.

3-10
C
Appl.
Impl.

Which of the following recommendations would be helpful to Judy in reducing her symptoms of PMS? Judy should:

a. take estrogen supplements.
b. avoid strenuous physical activity.
c. enroll in a program of aerobic exercises.
d. reduce salt intake and oral fluids.

3-11
D
Know.
Analy.

The physiological factor that is thought to be responsible for dysmenorrhea is an increase in the production of:

a. estrogen.
b. progesterone.
c. gonadotrophin-releasing hormone (GnRH).
d. prostaglandins.

Freda Johnston, a 47-year-old housewife, is complaining of "hot flashes" associated with menopause.

(THE FOLLOWING 5 ITEMS RELATE TO THE ABOVE PASSAGE.)

3-12
A
Know.
Asses.

The onset of menopause is directly related to the low levels of:

a. estrogen.
b. progesterone.
c. FSH.
d. LH.

3-13
A
Appl.
Impl.

Freda relates to the nurse that she fears something is going wrong inside her body because her sexual drives have increased recently. The nurse's best response would be:

a. "This is not an unusual happening. Many women report that they have an increased interest in sex during menopause."
b. "Most women report a decreased interest in sex during menopause; however, there is nothing wrong with your increased interest."
c. "Interest in sex is an individual desire; it is not associated with menopause."
d. "Women who were sexually active prior to menopause usually remain sexually active during and following menopause."

3-14
B
Appl.
Impl.

Freda tells the nurse she is experiencing discomfort during intercourse due to vaginal dryness. The nurse's best recommendation would be the use of:

a. petroleum jelly as a lubricant.
b. a water-soluble lubricant.
c. body cream or body lotion as a lubricant.
d. mild soap (castile) as a lubricant.

3-15
A
Appl.
Impl.

To help Freda in the psychological adjustment to menopause, the nurse should assist her in the development of a/an:

a. positive attitude toward her body.
b. acceptance of the fact that she is no longer a young woman.
c. positive attitude due to the fact that she can't get pregnant and sex can be less worrisome now.
d. interest in senior citizen groups where other women share her physiological problems.

3-16
B
Appl.
Asses.

The major reason the vulvular organs atrophy as a woman ages is that:

a. blood supply decreases.
b. hormonal activity decreases.
c. nerve impulses decrease.
d. sexual activity decreases.

3-17
D
Appl.
Analy.

The greatest influence on the child's attitudes concerning sex is his/her:

a. peers.
b. choice of movies, TV, and books.
c. church affiliation.
d. family and home environment.

3-18
C
Know.
Asses.

According to Masters and Johnson, the male ejaculates during which phase of sexual response?

a. excitement
b. plateau
c. orgasm
d. resolution

Jan Hillis, RN, is working in an OB-GYN clinic. Her main responsibility is to take a complete history from each client before that client is seen by the physician.

(THE FOLLOWING 3 ITEMS RELATE TO THE ABOVE PASSAGE.)

3-19
B
Appl.
Impl.

When taking a sexual history from a client, Jan should:

a. ask questions that require only "yes" or "no" answers.
b. ask open-ended questions.
c. write down everything the client says during the interview.
d. ignore the client's verbal remarks and concentrate on her nonverbal behavior during the interview.

3-20
A
Appl.
Impl.

During the client interview, Jan must obtain information concerning any history of sexually transmitted diseases. The best way for Jan to handle this subject is to:

a. make a general statement, then proceed to a more direct question.
b. ask direct questions to obtain the information she needs.
c. apologize for having to ask such personal questions.
d. let the physician complete that portion of the history.

3-21
B
Comp.
Impl.

In order for Jan to be an effective counselor concerning sexuality, she must first:

a. have in-depth knowledge about the client and her needs.
b. be aware of her own feelings, values, and attitudes toward sex.
c. be aware of her client's feelings, values, and attitudes toward sex.
d. complete an in-depth study of the sexual behaviors of humans.

3-22
D
Appl.
Impl.

In the event a client approaches a nurse about a problem concerning sexuality, and the nurse is not comfortable discussing sex, the nurse should:

a. handle the situation the best s/he can under the circumstances.
b. answer the questions asked, but not offer any additional information.
c. tell the client s/he is not comfortable discussing sexual matters.
d. refer the client to a nurse who is comfortable discussing sexual matters.

Amos King and Andrea Fisher are planning to be married in 3 months. They have come to the Health Department to discuss various methods of birth control with the family planning nurse.

(THE FOLLOWING 6 ITEMS RELATE TO THE ABOVE PASSAGE.)

3-23
D
Appl.
Impl.

Andrea asks the nurse, "What do you suggest as the best method of birth control?" The nurse's best reply would be:

a. "The best method of fertility control is the birth control pill."
b. "The various forms of mechanical contraceptives seem to be the most reliable methods of birth control."
c. "The intrauterine device (IUD) poses the least amount of problems and provides the greatest success rate for fertility control."
d. "A birth control method must meet your individual needs."

3-24
B
Appl.
Impl.

Andrea asks the nurse, "Can you explain to us how to use the basal body temperature method to detect ovulation and to prevent pregnancy?" The nurse's best reply to Andrea would be:

a. "Take your temperature every evening at the same time and keep a record for a period of several weeks. A noticeable drop in temperature indicates ovulation.
b. "Take your temperature every morning at the same time and keep a record of the findings. A noticeable rise in temperature indicates ovulation."
c. "Take your temperature at the same time each day and keep a record of each finding.
A noticeable drop in temperature indicates ovulation."
d. "This is an unscientific and unproven method of determining ovulation not recognized as a means of birth control."

3-25
D
Comp.
Analy.

The nurse tells Amos and Andrea that there are many choices concerning contraception. One choice that does not include the use of artificial devices or substances is the:

a. pill.
b. condom.
c. diaphragm.
d. basal body temperature method.

3-26
C
Appl.
Impl.

The nurse tells the couple that the use of the diaphragm is an excellent method of contraception provided the woman:

a. does not use any creams or jellies with it that might make it slip.
b. removes it promptly following intercourse and then douches.
c. leaves it in place for 6 hours following intercourse.
d. inserts it at least 4 hours prior to intercourse in order to form a protective seal.

3-27 The nurse tells the couple that the use of a condom is also a reliable method of
C   contraception provided:
Appl.
Impl.   a. the condom is applied immediately before ejaculation.
        b. the condom is applied tightly over the end of the penis to prevent ejaculation.
        c. the penis is withdrawn from the vagina while still erect and the rim of the
           condom is held to prevent the contents from spilling.
        d. the condom is applied before erection so it fits as snugly as possible.

3-28 Andrea asks the nurse about the effectiveness of "the pill" as a method of contraception.
A   The nurse should explain to Andrea that the pill:
Appl.
Impl.   a. is a very reliable method of contraception, but it may produce undesirable side
           effects.
        b. is only reliable as a method of contraception after one has taken it for at least
           3 months.
        c. has too many undesirable side effects that pose too great a risk for most women.
        d. is only effective if it is taken immediately before intercourse.

Jim and Dora Leigh have 4 children and have come to their physician's office to
discuss methods of sterilization.

(THE FOLLOWING 2 ITEMS RELATE TO THE ABOVE PASSAGE.)

3-29 During their initial interview by the nurse, Jim and Dora ask her/him what would be the
D   safest method of sterilization. The nurse replies, "Generally, the safest method of
Appl. sterilization would be a:
Impl.
        a. laparotomy."
        b. laparoscopy."
        c. minilaparotomy."
        d. vasectomy."

3-30 Jim asks the nurse if he will be sterile immediately following a vasectomy. The
C   nurse's best answer would be:
Appl.
Impl.   a. "You may still ejaculate live sperm for 4 to 6 months following a vasectomy."
        b. "You may ejaculate live sperm for 3 to 4 days following a vasectomy."
        c. "It takes 1 to 2 months and up to 36 ejaculations to clear the live sperm."
        d. "Immediate sterilization follows a successful vasectomy."

Lill Tish, a 35-year-old waitress, complains of pain, tenderness, and swelling in
both breasts that becomes more severe premenstrually. She has been examined
by her gynecologist and diagnosed as having bilateral fibrocystic breast disease.

(THE FOLLOWING 5 ITEMS RELATE TO THE ABOVE PASSAGE.)

3-31
A
Appl.
Asses.

When assessing Lill's breasts, the nurse finds palpable nodules which are similar in both breasts. Lill asks the nurse, "Can you tell by feeling if these nodules are benign or malignant?" The nurse's best reply concerning the differences between benign and malignant tumors would be:

a. "Cysts are usually well-circumscribed and movable, and there would be no retraction of the surrounding tissue. With a malignancy of this size, it probably would not be movable, and frequently there is retraction of the skin in the surrounding tissue."
b. "Cysts are irregular in shape and are not usually movable. When there is a malignancy, the mass has well-defined margins and is movable."
c. "With fibrocystic disease such as yours, there is pain, the cysts are large, solid, irregular masses, and there is always a discharge from the nipple. These characteristics are not present when there is a malignancy."
d. "It is impossible to distinguish a benign tumor from a malignant tumor by a physical evaluation. They feel basically the same."

3-32
B
Appl.
Asses.

To confirm the diagnosis of fibrocystic breast disease, the physician has ordered a mammogram. Lill asks, "What is a mammogram?" The nurse's best reply would be, "A mammogram is:

a. soft tissue radiography which visualizes breast tissue by the use of contrast media."
b. a non-painful, non-invasive, soft-tissue radiograph."
c. a method of visualizing the soft-tissue of the breast by using high doses of radiation."
d. a radiograph specific to the visualization of malignant tumors of the breast."

3-33
B
Appl.
Impl.

Lill asks the nurse if there is a possibility of her condition becoming malignant. The nurse's best reply would be:

a. "Once fibrocystic disease has invaded the breast tissue it is rare for a malignancy to occur."
b. "With fibrocystic disease there is an increased risk of developing breast cancer."
c. "There is no correlation between having fibrocystic disease and the development of cancer of the breast."
d. "Unless you get rid of your diseased breast tissue, it is 100% sure that you will develop cancer of the breast."

3-34
C
Appl.
Impl.

During the initial client interview, the nurse discovers Lill does not perform regular breast self-examinations (BSE). In addition to teaching Lill the proper technique of BSE, the nurse should also advise her as to how frequently the examinations be performed. The nurse's best response would be:

a. "BSE should be performed once a month just prior to the beginning of your menstrual period."
b. "BSE should be performed every month at the end of your menstrual period."
c. "BSE is to be performed every month about one week after your menstrual period."
d. "BSE must be performed every month immediately following ovulation."

3-35
D
Appl.
Impl.

Lill asks the nurse, "Is it necessary for me to perform regular breast self-examination? My breasts are so lumpy I don't know what I am feeling for. I would rather come and let you check my breasts periodically." The nurse's best reply would be:

a. "It will not be necessary for you to do regular breast self-examinations as long as you are faithful about coming to the office on a routine basis."
b. "With fibrocystic disease breast changes occur frequently. BSE should be done at least once a week to detect changes."
c. "I will be glad to come to your home and examine your breasts on a routine basis."
d. "It is important for you to perform periodic breast self-examinations. You know how your breasts feel, and you can detect any changes."

Viola Collins is a 53-year-old married housewife with 4 children. During BSE, Viola found a mass in the upper, outer quadrant of her left breast. She underwent a left breast biopsy 2 days ago in the outpatient surgery clinic, and the pathology report confirmed carcinoma of the breast. Viola is being admitted to the hospital for a left mastectomy.

(THE FOLLOWING 10 ITEMS RELATE TO THE ABOVE PASSAGE.)

3-36
C
Appl.
Impl.

During Viola's initial nursing assessment, the nurse notices Viola seems to be nervous and depressed about her impending surgery. The nurse should react to this by:

a. saying nothing, giving Viola the opportunity to express her feelings.
b. being cheerful and trying to get Viola to go to the dayroom to interact with other ambulatory patients.
c. encouraging Viola to ask questions and to express her feelings and concerns.
d. expressing sympathy over the fact that Viola will lose her breast, but including the positive statement that the surgery will save her life.

3-37
A
Comp.
Diag.

Viola looks at her breast and says, "This can't be happening to me. I just don't believe I have cancer and am going to lose my breast." Which phase of long-term adjustment does this represent?

a. shock phase
b. reaction phase
c. recovery phase
d. reorientation phase

3-38
B
Know.
Asses.

With the surgeon, Viola and her husband Jim discuss the various surgical procedures that can be performed to treat cancer of the breast. They agree to a modified radical mastectomy. This procedure involves the removal of:

a. all breast tissue, chest muscles, and axillary lymph nodes.
b. all breast tissue and axillary lymph nodes, while preserving the chest muscles.
c. internal breast tissue only.
d. the tumor and 2 to 3 cm of surrounding tissue.

3-39
A
Appl.
Impl.

Upon Viola's return to her room following surgery, the nurse takes her vital signs. The best way to take her blood pressure at this time is to use:

a. the right antecubital space.
b. the right popliteal area.
c. the left popliteal area.
d. a central venous pressure line.

3-40
C
Appl.
Impl.

To put Viola in a position of comfort, the nurse should:

a. elevate the left arm on a pillow and position the hand and elbow level with the shoulder.
b. abduct the left arm and position a pillow between the arm and the chest.
c. elevate the left arm on a pillow, position the hand higher than the elbow, and position the elbow higher than the shoulder.
d. keep the left arm flat on the bed dependent to the shoulder.

3-41
C
Appl.
Impl.

On Viola's third postop day, the nurse incorporates activities of daily living for therapeutic exercise. The nurse will encourage Viola to use her left hand and arm to:

a. brush her teeth.
b. button her bed jacket.
c. brush her hair.
d. squeeze a ball.

3-42
A
Appl.
Impl.

One of the interventions the nurse included on Viola's nursing care plan is "provide emotional support." The nurse can best do this by:

a. encouraging Viola to verbalize her fears and by answering her questions honestly.
b. discouraging her from talking about her surgery and diagnosis until she is able to cope better.
c. telling her that her surgery is over and that now she must look toward a positive future.
d. being sympathetic and telling Viola how brave she is for facing the problem and months of chemotherapy.

3-43
D
Appl.
Plan.

When planning Viola's postoperative care, emotional support is a number one priority. To be successful with this plan, the nurse MUST include the involvement of:

a. all health team members.
b. Viola's minister.
c. Viola's children.
d. Viola's husband.

3-44
A
Comp.
Impl.

Viola tells the nurse, "I have been thinking about having reconstructive breast surgery. What do you think?" Knowing that Viola's carcinoma was Stage I and that she underwent a modified radical mastectomy, the nurse should:

a. agree that Viola is a good candidate for reconstructive surgery.
b. suggest that Viola wait at least 5 years until she is sure she is free of cancer.
c. discourage thoughts about reconstructive surgery, knowing the type of mastectomy Viola underwent.
d. suggest Viola consult a plastic surgeon before discussing it with her husband and getting her hopes up.

3-45
D
Appl.
Asses.

One year following Viola's surgery she becomes a volunteer for the American Cancer Society's "Reach to Recovery" program. At this point Viola should be in which phase of the long-term adjustment period?

a. shock phase
b. reaction phase
c. recovery phase
d. reorientation phase

Jenny Long, a 27-year-old teacher, has been married for 1 year. She has been experiencing severe pelvic pain and dyspareunia. Her gynecologist performed a laparoscopy and diagnosed endometriosis.

(THE FOLLOWING 2 ITEMS RELATE TO THE ABOVE PASSAGE.)

3-46
C
Know.
Impl.

Since Jenny has indicated she would like to get pregnant, the expected treatment of her endometriosis would include:

a. progesterone.
b. antibiotics.
c. danazol.
d. estrogen.

3-47
D
Comp.
Asses.

In addition to the pain, one of the reasons many women with endometriosis seek medical care is due to the:

a. amenorrhea.
b. anovulatory cycle.
c. increased vaginal discharge.
d. infertility.

3-48
A
Appl.
Analy.

Fran Carson is being discharged from the hospital today. Her admitting diagnosis was toxic shock syndrome (TSS). During discharge planning, the nurse should tell Fran to:

a. use sanitary napkins and avoid the use of tampons.
b. use a diaphragm instead of a coil as a means of birth control.
c. limit sexual intercourse to only 1 or 2 safe partners.
d. have her partner wear a condom until she is no longer toxic.

3-49
B
Know.
Asses.

Terri Diggs has consulted her gynecologist about a severe vaginal itching. The physician has diagnosed the problem as monilial vaginitis. Factors that contribute to monilial vaginitis include the use of:

a. vaginal creams.
b. antibiotics.
c. large doses of vitamins.
d. circulatory stimulants.

3-50
A
Appl.
Impl.

Brenda Byrd is seeking medical treatment for a vaginal discharge. Her physician has diagnosed the problem as trichomoniasis and has prescribed metronidazole. The nurse is responsible for informing Brenda of the nursing implications of this drug. Her/his instructions should be:

a. "Both partners must be treated with the medication."
b. "Alcohol should be limited while taking this medication."
c. "It will turn you urine orange."
d. "It may produce drowsiness."

3-51
B
Know.
Asses.

The nurse knows that trichomoniasis is a sexually transmitted disease caused by a:

a. herpes zoster virus.
b. protozoan.
c. herpes simplex.
d. spirochete.

3-52
C
Comp.
Asses.

Regina Watkins has been admitted to the hospital with pelvic inflammatory disease (PID). The nurse will observe and assess Regina carefully because s/he knows it is not uncommon for a woman with PID to develop:

a. appendicitis.
b. cholecystitis.
c. salpingitis.
d. vulvitis.

3-53
A
Appl.
Impl.

Yvonne Martinez, a 50-year-old housewife with 6 children, is seeking medical care because of stress incontinence. The physician diagnoses her condition as being caused by a cystocele. One successful method of treating a cystocele is by performing Kegel exercises. The nurse teaches Yvonne to do these exercises by telling her to:

a. imagine she is voiding and then imagine she is stopping the flow of urine by tightening her pubococcygeal muscles.
b. wait to void as long as she can after she feels the urge to void in order to strengthen the pubococcygeal muscles.
c. increase her liquid intake, which will increase the daily contractions of both her bladder and pubococcygeal muscles.
d. do toe-touching and sit-up exercises daily to strengthen the abdominal and pelvic muscles.

Susan Hine shares with you that she has just been informed by her physician that, due to cervical cancer, she needs to have a hysterectomy. She appears upset and expresses a lack of knowledge regarding the procedure.

(THE FOLLOWING 4 ITEMS RELATE TO THE ABOVE PASSAGE.)

3-54
D
Comp.
Plan.

In order for Susan to make an informed decision to undergo the hysterectomy, she should be knowledgeable regarding:

a. the indications for having the surgery.
b. the effects of the surgery on childbearing ability and/or sexual performance.
c. the risks of the surgery.
d. all of these.

3-55
C
Know.
Diag.

A total hysterectomy involves the removal of:

a. the uterus, bilateral fallopian tubes, and bilateral ovaries.
b. unilateral or bilateral ovaries and fallopian tubes.
c. the uterus and cervical os.
d. the uterus and unilateral ovary and fallopian tube.

3-56
A
Appl.
Plan.

Routine postoperative care following Susan's abdominal hysterectomy will include:

a. checking the amount of bleeding by assessing the abdominal dressing.
b. assisting with sitz baths.
c. assisting with the heat lamp.
d. maintaining patency of the suprapubic catheter.

3-57
D
Know.
Asses.

The most frequently reported psychologic reaction after pelvic surgery, especially a hysterectomy, is:

a. anger.
b. fear.
c. frustration.
d. depression.

3-58
C
Know.
N/A

The largest group of people living below poverty level is:

a. adults in communal living situations.
b. young married couples under the age of 20.
c. single women with children.
d. single adults.

3-59
B
Know.
N/A

The increase in the number of female-headed households is closely associated with:

a. the Women's Movement.
b. divorce.
c. increased death rates among men.
d. the sexual revolution.

3-60   In general, as a result of divorce:
D
Know.   a. one's standard of living remains unchanged.
N/A   b. the male's standard of living decreases because of child support.
        c. both parties' standard of living decreases.
        d. the woman's standard of living decreases.

3-61   Which of the following is TRUE concerning custody of children in divorce cases?

Know.   a. The chance of getting custody is about equal for both parents.
Analy. b. Joint custody is usually awarded to both partners.
        c. Women receive custody in a greater number of cases.
        d. The courts tend to retain custody of the child.

3-62   The labor market is associated with women and poverty for all of the following reasons
B   EXCEPT:
Comp.
Analy. a. there are few job opportunities open to women.
        b. women often occupy low-paid positions.
        c. women have jobs that have less unionization.
        d. there are fewer job benefits in positions occupied by women.

3-63   Which of the following is TRUE of the welfare system?
B
Comp.   a. The amount of assistance usually exceeds the poverty level.
Analy. b. The welfare system eliminates work incentives.
        c. There is no cap on earnings that a family can take in.
        d. A cost of living increase is included each year.

3-64   Funding cuts have adversely affected those living in poverty. All of the following
A   programs have had cutbacks EXCEPT:
Know.
N/A   a. health insurance providers.
        b. food stamp programs.
        c. aid to families with dependent children (AFDC).
        d. women, infants, and children (WIC) nutrition program.

3-65   Sally Drummond is a single parent who is pregnant with her third child. During her
D   initial visit to the prenatal clinic, Sally tells you she cannot afford to stay on the diet
Appl.   you have described. The most appropriate nursing intervention is to:
Impl.
        a. show her a film about good nutrition in pregnancy.
        b. discuss the option of abortion.
        c. tell her that the fetus requires adequate maternal nutrition.
        d. assist Sally in finding a community resource that could help in providing food.

3-66   Pregnant women working in the lead industry may have all of the following adverse
A   effects EXCEPT:
Comp.
Diag.   a. abruptio placenta.
        b. spontaneous abortion.
        c. stillbirth.
        d. premature birth.

3-67
D
Know. Reproductive problems may be associated with exposure to:
Diag.
    a. antineoplastic drugs.
    b. pesticides.
    c. anesthetic gases.
    d. all of these.

3-68
D
Know. The person who rapes may be:
Diag.
    a. a stranger.
    b. an acquaintance.
    c. a husband.
    d. any of these.

3-69
D
Know. Legally, all of the following are preconditions for a valid charge of rape EXCEPT:
Diag.
    a. nonconsent of the victim.
    b. coitus or vaginal penetration, however slight.
    c. the use of threat, physical force, deception, or intimidation.
    d. witness, by the victim, of the presence of a weapon.

3-70
B
Know. The most appropriate definition of rape is:
Diag.
    a. a violent act of sex.
    b. an act of violence expressed sexually.
    c. an act of sex utilized to deal with feelings of depression.
    d. an act of sex for the purpose of increasing one's perception of self-worth.

Cindy Reed comes to the crisis prevention center anxious and upset. She informs the volunteer nurse that she has been raped.

(THE FOLLOWING 2 ITEMS RELATE TO THE ABOVE PASSAGE.)

3-71
B
Appl. Cindy states, "I think it is probably my fault this happened. I should never have worn that tight skirt." Which response by the nurse would be most appropriate?
Impl.
    a. "You should not dwell on why it happened. Now you need to deal with the complications that may occur because of the rape."
    b. "Your reaction represents a myth. Women do not have to provoke the assailant to be raped."
    c. "You need to begin to refrain from blaming yourself."
    d. "Even if you did provoke the assailant by wearing a tight skirt, he is responsible for his behavior."

3-72
C
Appl. Cindy informs the nurse that she does not know the person who raped her and that she had never seen him prior to the event. She adds, "What kind of person would do a thing like this?" All of the following would be appropriate responses EXCEPT:
Impl.
    a. "More than half of the rapists are under 25 years of age."
    b. "3 out of 5 rapists are married."
    c. "Most rapists experience sexual difficulties in their day-to-day lives."
    d. "Rapists come from all ethnic backgrounds."

Mary Flowers has been attending support group meetings at the rape crisis center since she was raped 2 months ago.

(THE FOLLOWING 3 ITEMS RELATE TO THE ABOVE PASSAGE.)

3-73
A
Appl.
Plan.

The nurse who leads the support group is familiar with the many different responses of victims. All of the following are true EXCEPT:

a. rape is often viewed as a developmental crisis.
b. the victim is generally unprepared to handle the event.
c. the victim experiences disequilibrium and loss of control.
d. A crisis state does not necessarily follow rape; some victims can avoid the crisis.

3-74
A
Comp.
Diag.

After a rape, the victim's crisis response develops in three stages. Accurate information regarding these stages includes:

a. the victim utilizes habitual problem-solving techniques to cope with the crisis.
b. stress and discomfort decrease with each passing day.
c. the victim mobilizes her internal and external resources to solve her problem, and this increases her anxiety.
d. recovery depends on the victim's ability to forget the incident.

3-75
A
Know.
Plan.

The goal of the outward adjustment phase is:

a. to provide the victim a means of regaining control of her life.
b. to provide the victim time to express her feelings through physical manifestations.
c. to provide the victim a means of resolving her emotional trauma.
d. all of these.

Chapter 4

Families with Special Reproductive Problems

Instructions: For each of the following multiple-choice questions, select the ONE most appropriate answer.

Dan and Rose McCarty have been married for 3 years. They have been trying to have a baby for the past 2 years, but Rose has been unable to conceive. They are in the physician's office to be evaluated for infertility.

(THE FOLLOWING 9 ITEMS RELATE TO THE ABOVE PASSAGE.)

4-1
D
Know.
Asses.

An analysis of Dan's ejaculate proves sperm count to be within normal limits. This would mean that Dan's sperm is equal to or greater in number than _____ per ml.

a. 5,000
b. 50,000
c. 500,000
d. 5,000,000

4-2
B
Know.
Asses.

The BASIC assessment to monitor ovulation in Rose would be:

a. an ovarian biopsy.
b. the basal body temperature recording.
c. a cervical biopsy.
d. a pelvic x-ray.

4-3
C
Appl.
Plan.

The physician wants to evaluate the patency of Rose's fallopian tubes. A hysterosalpingogram is the test of choice. The nurse tells Rose this will be done:

a. just prior to her menstrual period.
b. during her menstrual period.
c. prior to ovulation.
d. immediately following ovulation.

4-4
C
Appl.
Plan.

Rose asks the nurse, "Is a hysterosalpingogram painful?" The nurse's best reply would be:

a. "There is no pain associated with a hysterosalpingogram."
b. "You will be asleep for the procedure and will feel nothing at all."
c. "You may have some gas-like pains in your abdomen and may feel pain in your shoulder when you sit up."
d. "You may have some abdominal pain and pain in the area of your diaphragm, but you should not experience severe pain."

4-5
C
Appl.
Eval.

A postcoital examination is to be performed. The nurse tells Rose, "The purpose of this test it to determine:

a. the quantity of viable sperm that are ejaculated."
b. the quality of viable sperm that are ejaculated."
c. the sperm's ability to survive the cervical barrier."
d. the presence of either an alkaline or acidic environment."

4-6
A
Know.
Diag.

Rose, who has never conceived, is diagnosed as having:

a. primary infertility.
b. secondary infertility.
c. psychological infertility.
d. physiological infertility.

4-7
B
Comp.
Plan.

To maximize their potential for fertilization, the nurse tells Dan and Rose they should engage in intercourse:

a. every night.
b. 1 to 3 times a week.
c. only once a week.
d. twice a day if possible.

4-8
C
Appl.
Impl.

The nurse tells Rose that her position following intercourse will help facilitate fertilization. S/he recommends that Rose remain in bed in a recumbent position for:

a. 10 minutes following intercourse.
b. 30 minutes following intercourse.
c. 1 hour following intercourse.
d. 2 to 3 hours following intercourse.

4-9
B
Appl.
Asses.

The nurse working with Dan and Rose knows the most difficult aspect of their problem is the:

a. financial aspect.
b. emotional aspect.
c. painful and time-consuming testing.
d. decision to adopt or remain childless.

Arthur Kerns, 41 years old, and Sue Kerns, 39 years old, have been married 9 years. After many years of trying to have a child, Sue did conceive. Because of her age, an amniocentesis was performed during the 16th week of gestation. The diagnosis of Down syndrome was made.

(THE FOLLOWING 5 ITEMS RELATE TO THE ABOVE PASSAGE.)

4-10
D
Appl.
Asses.

Because of her age, Sue is considered to be at greater risk than a younger woman for having a child with Down syndrome. At what age does the risk for chromosome abnormalities become a concern for women?

a. 30 years of age
b. 32 years of age
c. 35 years of age
d. 37 years of age

4-11
D
Appl.
Asses.

Before the amniocentesis was performed, Sue wanted to know why it was being done. The nurse explained that prenatal diagnostic testing, such as an amniocentesis, is performed to:

a. guarantee the birth of a normal child.
b. abort pregnancies in which the fetus has genetic abnormalities.
c. begin early treatment of an affected fetus.
d. detect abnormalities of the fetus.

4-12
A
Know.
Asses.

Down syndrome is an example of:

a. an autosome abnormality.
b. a sex chromosome abnormality.
c. an autosome plus sex chromosome abnormality.
d. either an autosome or a sex chromosome abnormality.

4-13
C
Appl.
Asses.

When the infant with Down syndrome is born, the nursery nurse assesses him for common dermatoglyphic patterns associated with this condition. These include:

a. a decreased number of ulnar loops, 3 to 4 creases in the palm, and a whorl pattern on the hallucal area of the foot.
b. no visible loops on the finger tips, multiple creases in the palm, and several ulnar loops on the toes.
c. a simian line in the palm, increased numbers of ulnar loops, and an arch tibial pattern on the hallucal area of the foot.
d. lack of visible lines in the palm of the hand, an increase in radial loops on the finger tips, and an increased whorl on the hallucal area of the foot.

4-14
D
Comp.
Asses.

A karyotype of the baby's chromosomes shows a trisomy 21. The nurse knows that the life expectancy for children with this condition is approximately:

a. 3 months.
b. 3 years.
c. 10 to 20 years.
d. 50 to 60 years.

Polly Wright, RN, works as a staff nurse in the nursery of a large metropolitan hospital. Polly specializes in caring for infants who are born with genetic/ chromosomal abnormalities.

(THE FOLLOWING 3 ITEMS RELATE TO THE ABOVE PASSAGE.)

4-15
A
Comp.
Impl.

A newborn female was admitted to the nursery with an order to send a specimen of the newborn's secretions to the lab to determine the presence of Barr bodies. Polly will take the specimen from the:

a. buccal area.
b. vaginal area.
c. sublingual area.
d. conjunctival area.

4-16 The number of Barr bodies found in a female child should be:
B
Know.   a. 0.
Asses.   b. 1.
          c. 4.
          d. 46.

4-17 A normal female karyotype consists of:
B
Comp.   a. 44 autosomes and two Y sex chromosomes.
Asses.   b. 44 autosomes and two X sex chromosomes.
          c. 44 autosomes plus one X and one Y sex chromosome.
          d. 46 autosomes plus one X and one Y sex chromosome.

John and Judy Taylor have been married for 2 years. John's father has Huntington's chorea and John is exhibiting mild symptoms of the disorder. John and Judy decide to visit a genetic counselor to discuss the risk of their having a baby with Huntington's chorea.

(THE FOLLOWING 3 ITEMS RELATE TO THE ABOVE PASSAGE.)

4-18 The counselor correctly informs John and Judy that Huntington's chorea is an
C   example of autosomal dominant inheritance, and there is:
Appl.
Impl.   a. no possibility of the affected male passing an abnormal gene to his offspring since this abnormal gene is carried by the female.
          b. approximately a 10% chance that the abnormal gene will be passed on to the offspring.
          c. as high as a 50% possibility that the abnormal gene will be passed on to the offspring.
          d. a 100% certainty that the affected parent will transmit the abnormal gene to the offspring.

4-19 To assist John and Judy in understanding the transmission of an autosomal dominant
D   inheritance, the counselor constructs a graphic representation for them. This graphic
Appl. representation is called a:
Plan.
          a. karyotype.
          b. family graph.
          c. genetic graph.
          d. family pedigree.

4-20 To eliminate the possibility of transmitting Huntington's chorea to their offspring,
A   John and Judy consider artificial insemination using:
Appl.
Plan.   a. donor sperm, implanted in Judy.
          b. John's sperm, implanted in a surrogate mother.
          c. John's sperm, implanted in Judy after genetic restructuring.
          d. donor sperm, implanted in John's sterilized testes.

Walter and Debra Scott's daughter, Tammy, is diagnosed as having cystic fibrosis. During their research on cystic fibrosis, they have learned it is a condition of autosomal recessive inheritance.

(THE FOLLOWING 2 ITEMS RELATE TO THE ABOVE PASSAGE.)

4-21
C
Appl.
Asses.

The nurse knows Tammy most likely inherited the disease from:

 a. her mother.
 b. her father.
 c. both parents, who are carriers of the abnormal gene.
 d. none of these.

4-22
D
Comp.
Asses.

Walter and Debra know that of any future children they decide to have:

 a. only the female children will be affected by the abnormal gene.
 b. all of them will be affected with cystic fibrosis.
 c. it is unlikely that any other children will be affected.
 d. there is a 25% chance of passing the abnormal gene to a child.

4-23
C
Comp.
Diag.

Mr. and Mrs. Thompson have a son, Johnny, who has been diagnosed as having muscular dystrophy. They also have a daughter, Amy, who is clinically well. They ask the pediatric nurse practitioner if there is a possibility that Amy will transmit muscular dystrophy to her offspring. The nurse's best response is:

 a. "Amy cannot pass the abnormal gene to her offspring since she does not have muscular dystrophy."
 b. "Amy cannot pass the abnormal gene to her male offspring, but she may pass it to her female offspring."
 c. "There is a 50% chance that Amy is a carrier and will pass the abnormal gene to her offspring."
 d. "Amy is definitely a carrier of the abnormal gene."

4-24
A
Comp.
Asses.

The genetic mechanism of diabetes mellitus is thought to be due to a/an:

 a. multifactorial, inheritance trait.
 b. X-linked, dominant, inheritance trait.
 c. autosomal, dominant, inheritance trait.
 d. autosomal, recessive, inheritance trait.

4-25
C
Comp.
Asses.

Sickle cell anemia, a condition that is not uncommon in the black population, is an example of a/an:

 a. multifactorial, inherited disorder.
 b. X-linked, recessive, inherited disorder.
 c. autosomal, recessive, inherited disorder.
 d. autosomal, dominant, inherited disorder.

PART 2

PREGNANCY

Chapter 5

Conception and Fetal Development

Instructions: For each of the following multiple-choice questions, select the ONE most appropriate answer.

5-1
D
Know.
Diag.

The unique characteristics of an individual are determined genetically by:

a. deoxyribonucleic acid (DNA).
b. ribonucliec acid (RNA).
c. chromosomes.
d. genes.

5-2
A
Know.
N/A

The chromosomal structure of human beings consists of:

a. 46 chromosomes: 22 pairs of autosomes and 1 pair of sex chromosomes.
b. 42 chromosomes: 20 pairs of autosomes and 1 pair of sex chromosomes.
c. 46 chromosomes: 20 pairs of autosomes and 2 pairs of sex chromosomes.
c. 40 chromosomes: 18 pairs of autosomes and 2 pairs of sex chromosomes.

Linda Epperson, RN, a nurse midwife, has been asked to speak to a local high school girls' club on conception and fetal development. She is now researching and reviewing pertinent material to cover in the presentation.

(THE FOLLOWING 9 ITEMS RELATE TO THE ABOVE PASSAGE.)

5-3
D
Appl.
Plan.

As Linda prepares her presentation for the class, she should include all of the following information EXCEPT:

a. females have 2 X chromosomes.
b. Males have X and Y chromosomes.
c. to produce a male the mother must contribute an X chromosome and the father a Y chromosome.
d. to produce a female, the mother must contribute 2 X chromosomes.

5-4
B
Appl.
Impl.

In explaining how fertilization occurs, which of the following would be the most accurate information?

a. The process of fertilization occurs in the upper third of the fallopian tube.
b. High estrogen levels during ovulation help move the ovum down the fallopian tube to be fertilized.
c. The process of fertilization occurs in the upper portion of the uterus.
d. The high estrogen levels during ovulation cause thickening of the cervical mucus, which facilitates penetration by the sperm.

5-5   The transmission of potential hereditary characteristics is the function of the:
C
Know.   a. amnion.
N/A   b. chromosomes.
         c. genes.
         d. gametes.

5-6   Linda should also include in her lecture the fact that transportation of the zygote
A   through the fallopian tube into the cavity of the uterus takes a minimum of:
Appl.
Plan.   a. 3 days.
         b. 12 hours.
         c. 18 hours.
         d. 5 days.

5-7   The blastocyst implants itself in the uterine lining approximately _____ days
C   after fertilization.
Appl.
Asses.   a. 1
         b. 2 to 4
         c. 7 to 9
         d. 21

5-8   The embryonic membranes begin to form at the time of implantation. The purpose
A   of these membranes is to:
Know.
Diag.   a. protect and support the embryo.
         b. cushion the embryo against mechanical injury.
         c. provide a means of metabolic and nutrient exchange.
         d. provide red blood cells.

5-9   Linda should also explain to the group that the first membrane to form is the
C   _____, the outermost embryonic membrane.
Appl.
Impl.   a. amnion
         b. amniotic sac
         c. chorion
         d. mesoderm

5-10   True placental formation begins:
C
Know.   a. at conception.
Analy.   b. during the time of implantation.
         c. during the third week of gestation.
         d. during the third month of gestation.

5-11   The placenta is divided into segments called:
A
Know.   a. cotyledons.
Analy.   b. decidua.
         c. syncytium.
         d. villi.

Linda has concluded her presentation to the girls' club. She has asked for questions from the group to clarify any misunderstanding of the material or misinformation the girls may have.

(THE FOLLOWING 5 ITEMS RELATE TO THE ABOVE PASSAGE.)

5-12
C
Comp.
Diag.

A member of the club asks Linda to explain the functions of the amniotic fluid. All of the following responses are CORRECT EXCEPT:

a. to cushion against mechanical injury.
b. to control the embryo's temperature.
c. to provide a means of nutrient exchange for the embryo/fetus.
d. to allow freedom of movement so the embryo/fetus can change position.

5-13
C
Know.
Asses.

After 20 weeks, the volume of amniotic fluid is:

a. 200 to 600 mL.
b. 350 to 500 mL.
c. 500 to 1000 mL.
d. 1000 to 1500 mL.

5-14
A
Analy.
Know.

Another question raised is, "How many vessels are there normally in the umbilical cord?" Linda's best response is:

a. 1 vein and 2 arteries.
b. 2 veins and 1 artery.
c. 1 vein and 1 artery.
d. 2 veins and 2 arteries.

5-15
B
Asses.
Know.

Which of the following would be typical of a fetus at 20 weeks?

a. The fetus has a body weight of 780 gms.
b. The fetus actively sucks and swallows amniotic fluid.
c. Formation of urine begins.
d. Lanugo is disappearing.

5-16
A
Appl.
Asses.

"Can you tell us about the baby's heart?" Linda replies, "The heart of the embryo is a distinguishable organ by the _____ week of development."

a. 8th
b. 14th
c. 17th
d. 24th

Jackie Robbins is 24 years old and 7 months pregnant. She has come to the obstetrical clinic for a routine prenatal examination. She is very anxious because she spontaneously aborted during her last pregnancy.

(THE FOLLOWING 3 QUESTIONS RELATE TO THE ABOVE PASSAGE.)

5-17
A
Appl.
Diag.

During Jackie's assessment, the nurse hears a soft blowing sound over the location of the fetus' umbilical cord. The rate of the sound is synchronous with the fetal heartbeat. The nurse identifies this as:

a. a normal sound called funic souffle.
b. an abnormal sound representing an aortic aneurysm.
c. a normal sound called Wharton's tone.
d. an abnormal sound representing a false knot in the cord.

5-18
D
Comp.
Asses.

The placenta produces hormones that are vital to the function of the fetus. Which hormone is PRIMARILY responsible for the maintenance of pregnancy past the 11th week?

a. human chorionic gonadotropin (hCG)
b. human placental lactogen (hPL)
c. testosterone
d. progesterone

5-19
B
Comp.
Impl.

Jackie is curious about the function of the lungs in the fetus. She asks the nurse, "How does the baby get air?" The nurse would give Jackie good information in each of the following responses EXCEPT:

a. "The lungs of the fetus do not carry out respiratory gas exchange in utero."
b. "The blood from the placenta is carried through the umbilical artery, which penetrates the abdominal wall of the fetus."
c. "The placenta assumes the function of the fetal lungs by supplying oxygen and allowing the excretion of carbon dioxide into the maternal bloodstream."
d. "The fetus is able to obtain sufficient oxygen due to the fact that the hemoglobin concentration in the fetus is about 50% greater than that of the mother."

Paula Cartwright, RN, is a part-time labor and delivery nurse. She has been asked by an obstetrician to plan and implement prenatal classes for her/his clients. Paula decides to include the following information on embryo/fetal development and organ formation.

(THE FOLLOWING 7 ITEMS RELATE TO THE ABOVE PASSAGE.)

5-20
B
Know.
Asses.

The post-conception age of the newborn is usually:

a. 32 weeks.
b. 38 weeks.
c. 40 weeks.
d. 44 weeks.

5-21
B
Know.
Asses.

The embryo's arm and leg buds are well developed and the brain is differentiated by the the _____ week.

a. 3rd
b. 4th to 5th
c. 6th
d. 9th to 12th

5-22 At the _____ week, the embryo is approximately 1.2 inches long, the external
A genitals are visible, and long bones are beginning to form.
Comp.
Asses. a. 8th
  b. 16th
  c. 24th
  d. 28th

5-23 During the _____ week, the brain is developing rapidly and the nervous
B system is complete enough to provide some regulation of body function.
Know.
Asses. a. 17th to 20th
  b. 25th to 28th
  c. 29th to 32nd
  d. 33rd to 36th

5-24 At the end of the _____ week, the embryo is sufficiently developed to be called
A a fetus.
Know.
Analy. a. 8th
  b. 12th
  c. 18th
  d. 22nd

5-25 The fragile blood vessels of the umbilical cord are not compressed by the pressure
B of the uterus since the vessels are protected by:
Asses.
Appl. a. a cushion of amniotic fluid.
  b. a padding of Wharton's jelly.
  c. a thick muscle layer.
  d. highly absorbent vessel walls.

5-26 Identify the INCORRECT statement regarding twins.
C
Appl. a. Despite their birth relationship, fraternal twins are no more similar to each other
Diag.   than they would be if they had been born singly.
  b. Fraternal twins may be the same or different sex.
  c. Identical twins occur more frequently than fraternal twins.
  d. Congenital abnormalities are more prevalent in identical twins.

5-27 Following the release of the ovum from the ovary, the maximum time in which
A fertilization can occur is:
Comp.
Asses. a. 24 hours.
  b. 36 hours.
  c. 48 hours.
  d. 72 hours.

Chapter 6

Physical and Psychological Changes of Pregnancy

Instructions: For each of the following multiple-choice questions, select the ONE most appropriate answer.

Linda White, at 24 weeks' gestation, comes to the prenatal clinic for her regularly scheduled appointment.

(THE FOLLOWING 10 ITEMS RELATE TO THE ABOVE PASSAGE.)

6-1
C
Comp.
Asses.

In assessing Linda, the nurse should keep in mind that during pregnancy the blood pressure normally:

a. remains constant.
b. increases gradually.
c. reaches prepregnant levels at term.
d. is dramatically affected by fetal activity.

6-2
C
Know.
Asses.

Which one of the following changes occurs in the organ systems of Linda's body as a result of the pregnancy?

a. The uterus doubles in size.
b. The cervix becomes more pale and firm.
c. Nosebleeds (epistaxis) and nasal stiffness may occur.
d. Gastric emptying time increases.

6-3
A
Appl.
Diag.

The nurse notes that Linda's blood pressure prior to the pregnancy was 118/68. An expected blood pressure for Linda on this visit would be:

a. 98/60.
b. 118/68.
c. 120/80.
d. 148/84.

6-4
B
Know.
Impl.

The nurse instructs Linda to rest in a side-lying position and avoid lying flat on her back. The nurse explains that this is to avoid "vena caval syndrome," a condition which:

a. occurs when blood pressure increases sharply with changes in position.
b. results when blood flow from the extremities is blocked or slowed.
c. is seen mainly in first pregnancies.
d. may require medication if positioning does not help.

6-5
A
Comp.
Diag.

During pregnancy the plasma volume increases to a greater extent than the number of red blood cells. This change results in:

a. pseudo-anemia.
b. physiologic leukocytosis.
c. blood which clots more readily.
d. varicosities in the lower extremities.

6-6
D
Appl.
Impl.

Linda complains that during her first few months of pregnancy it seemed like she "had to go to the bathroom every five minutes." The nurse explained that this was because:

a. she probably had a kidney infection.
b. bladder capacity normally increases throughout pregnancy.
c. women are often more preoccupied with body functions during pregnancy.
d. the growing uterus puts pressure on the bladder.

6-7
B
Know.
Analy.

In pregnancy, the glomerular filtration rate:

a. is directly influenced by the woman's posture.
b. increases significantly above prepregnanat levels.
c. makes the most dramatic changes near birth.
d. only changes when pathological conditions are present.

6-8
D
Appl.
Impl.

Linda tells the nurse that her sister developed large brown spots on her cheeks during pregnancy. Linda asks what other skin changes she might expect to see in her pregnancy. The nurse tells Linda that she might notice a:

a. lightening of the nipples and areola of the breasts.
b. marked decrease in sweating.
c. noticeable increase in the growth of her hair.
d. darkening of the abdominal midline from the pubic symphysis to the umbilicus.

6-9
B
Appl.
Impl.

The nurse does a dipstick analysis for glucose on a sample of Linda's urine and records a finding of "trace." Linda asks what "trace" means. The nurse replies:

a. "The doctor will talk to you about this later."
b. "This commonly means the kidneys are not able to keep up with reabsorbing all the glucose."
c. "You may be developing gestational diabetes."
d. "You will need to increase your exercise in order to avoid glucose wastage."

6-10
D
Know.
Diag.

Of the hormones produced during pregnancy, which one is MOST significant in maintaining the pregnancy?

a. human chorionic gonadotropin
b. human placental lactogen
c. estrogen
d. progesterone

Rita Collins, 22 years old, is 10 weeks pregnant with her first baby.

(THE FOLLOWING 5 ITEMS RELATE TO THE ABOVE PASSAGE.)

6-11
A
Comp.
Analy.

Rita complains of being nauseated periodically throughout the day for the past two weeks. The nurse understands that this is a common finding in early pregnancy PRIMARILY due to:

a. increased levels of hCG.
b. unconscious rejection of the fetus.
c. cultural expectations found mainly in Western societies.
d. sluggish intestinal peristalsis.

6-12
D
Appl.
Impl.

Rita also comments that she seems to be urinating more often. The nurse explains that frequent urination in early pregnancy is usually caused by:

a. fetal activity.
b. urinary tract infections.
c. excitement about the pregnancy.
d. bladder pressure from the enlarging uterus.

6-13
C
Know.
Analy.

As Rita's pregnancy progresses, probable signs of her pregnancy appear. Probable signs of pregnancy are:

a. subjective.
b. diagnostic of pregnancy.
c. observable by the examiner.
d. usually uncomfortable for the expectant mother.

6-14
A
Comp.
Analy.

Which of the following is a probable sign of pregnancy that Rita might be expected to have?

a. a bluish discoloration of the vagina and cervix
b. amenorrhea
c. fetal heart tones
d. morning sickness

6-15
B
Know.
Asses.

The nurse is usually able to first feel fetal movements on abdominal palpatation:

a. at 12 weeks.
b. around 20 weeks.
c. about 28 weeks.
d. near term.

Heather Chisolm, 19 years old, comes to the clinic after missing two menstrual periods to find out if she is pregnant.

(THE FOLLOWING 4 ITEMS RELATE TO THE ABOVE PASSAGE.)

6-16
D
Appl.
Impl.

A Gravidex pregnancy test is carried out, and Heather asks for information about the test. The nurse replies, "Pregnancy tests, based on immunoassay such as the Gravidex:

a. take about one week to obtain the results."
b. are the most accurate pregnancy tests available today."
c. require no special methods for collecting the test urine sample."
d. detect positive results 10 to 14 days after the first missed period."

6-17
A
Comp.
Analy.

In order to make an early positive diagnosis of pregnancy, the care provider might use ultrasound to:

a. detect the gestational sac.
b. hear the fetal heartbeat.
c. identify the placental souffle.
d. recognize the signs of vasocongestion in the uterus.

6-18
A
Appl.
Analy.

Which of the following behaviors would be a typical response in the first trimester of pregnancy that the nurse might see in Heather?

a. careful monitoring of changes in her body
b. daydreaming about how the baby will look and act after it is born
c. asking her friends about their experiences with childbirth
d. expressing concern about how she will act in labor

6-19
C
Appl.
Plan.

A variety of emotional responses normally occur throughout pregnancy. Which of the following comments by Heather might raise concerns in the nurse and warrant further assessment?

a. "I can't believe I'm pregnant."
b. "We've wanted children, but I wish my husband could have finished college first."
c. "I never wanted this baby."
d. "I'm as big as a barn. I feel so ugly."

Ellen Hubbard is a 21-year-old primigravida in the first trimester of pregnancy. She comes to the clinic for her second prenatal visit.

(THE FOLLOWING 2 ITEMS RELATE TO THE ABOVE PASSAGE.)

6-20
A
Appl.
Plan.

Following her prenatal examination, Ellen asks the nurse to recommend 1 or 2 good books for her to read on pregnancy and childbirth. The nurse recognizes this activity will help Ellen accomplish which of the following tasks of pregnancy?

a. Safe passage of the fetus.
b. Acceptance of the unborn child.
c. Committing herself to mothering the infant.
d. Learning to accept her body in its present condition.

41

6-21
C
Appl.
Impl.

On a subsequent prenatal visit, Ellen and Charles discuss their new roles as parents with the nurse. Charles comments that he really wants to be a good father to their new baby. The nurse explains that in developing the fatherhood role the most important thing is to:

a. participate actively in as many aspects of childbearing and childrearing as possible.
b. develop a role similar to that of his closest friend.
c. decide on a role that is mutually agreeable to both him and Ellen.
d. begin by following the basic pattern of fathering that his father used in raising him.

Theresa McCallister, 26 years old, is 20 weeks pregnant. She has a 1 & 1/2 -year-old son named Jeffery at home.

(THE FOLLOWING 2 ITEMS RELATE TO THE ABOVE PASSAGE.)

6-22
B
Appl.
Impl.

During her prenatal visit, Theresa asks the nurse how she should prepare her son Jeffery for the new baby. The nurse's best response would be:

a. "Introduce the baby to Jeffery initially when you bring the baby home from the hospital."
b. "Begin several weeks before the baby is due; let Jeffery feel the baby move inside your uterus."
c. "Jeffery should be included in every aspect of the pregnancy so that he will not feel excluded."
d. "Initiate an explanation of your pregnancy soon rather than waiting for Jeffery to ask questions."

6-23
B
Appl.
Eval.

Following an extensive discussion of sibling rivalry, the nurse asks Theresa to give some examples of how Jeffery might be expected to behave when the new baby is brought home. An appropriate response by Theresa would be:

a. "He will ignore the new baby since he's really too young to understand what's going on."
b. "He may want a to have a bottle or to climb into the baby's crib."
c. "He will be thrilled that he now has a new brother or sister to play with."
d. "He will feel important when I ask him to watch the baby while I do the dishes."

6-24
B
Appl.
Plan.

Maria Ochoa, a 23-year-old Philippine American, is 18 weeks pregnant. After receiving a prescription for prenatal vitamins, she tells the nurse that her mother always warned her not to take any medications during pregnancy. The nurse's initial intervention should be to:

a. remind Maria that the vitamins were ordered for her by the nurse midwife.
b. determine how important Maria's mother's advice is to her.
c. assure Maria that the pills are only vitamins and are not considered medication.
d. explain to Maria that without the vitamins her expected baby's growth and development could be endangered.

42

6-25   Ethnocentrism is the belief that:
C
Know.   a. cultural values are major determiners of one's behavior.
Analy. b. every cultural group has a core of beliefs which are common to every other
            culture.
        c. values and practices of one's own culture are superior.
        d. one can only see another's culture through the eyes of his/her own culture.

6-26   The nurse recognizes that pregnancy is a maturational crisis. Which of the following
A   primigravidas would be at risk for having the greatest difficulty resolving this crisis?
Appl.
Analy. a. Alice Green, 19 years old, who has just moved to the city with her husband
            Bob, also 19, from their hometown 1300 miles away.
        b. Sue Johnson, a 22-year-old single woman, who lives in a small apartment next
            to her mother.
        c. Ann Davis, 23 years old, whose husband Bill, 25 years old, has just been
            promoted to manager of a large grocery store.
        d. Phyllis Goodwin, 25 years old, who had been trying with her husband Ed, 26
            years old, for the past 4 years to conceive a child.

Chapter 7

Antepartal Nursing Assessment

Instructions: For each of the following multiple-choice questions, select the ONE most appropriate answer.

Anita Downing, 22 years old, comes to the clinic for her first prenatal examination.

(THE FOLLOWING 5 ITEMS RELATE TO THE ABOVE PASSAGE.)

7-1
B
Appl.
Plan.

The most important information that Anita should learn from this initial appointment is:

a. the nurse will help her find the best childbirth classes to attend.
b. it is important for her to keep her next clinic appointment.
c. no medications or alcohol should be consumed for the remainder of the pregnancy.
d. Anita's partner is always welcome at her appointments.

7-2
A
Appl.
Analy.

In giving the obstetrical history, Anita tells the nurse that she has been pregnant twice before. She had a miscarriage with the first pregnancy after 8 weeks. With the second pregnancy, she delivered twin girls at 34 weeks' gestation, but the babies died two days after birth. The nurse records Anita as being:

a. Gravida 3 Para 1.
b. Gravida 3 Para 0.
c. Gravida 3 Para 2.
d. Gravida 3 Para 2.

7-3
C
Know.
Asses.

Anita notices that the nurse has written the word "multigravida" in her chart and she asks the nurse what it means. The nurse replies, "Multigravida means:

a. pregnancy."
b. the first weeks of gestation."
c. a woman experiencing her second or more pregnancy."
d. a woman who has had two or more births at more than 20 weeks' gestation."

7-4
A
Appl.
Analy.

Using the TPAL system to record Anita's obstetrical history, the nurse should record:

a. Gravida 3 Para 0210.
b. Gravida 2 Para 2012.
c. Gravida 3 Para 0110.
d. Gravida 2 Para 1100.

7-5
A
Appl.
Eval.

The nurse and Anita discuss cigarette smoking and pregnancy. Following the discussion, the nurse asks Anita to explain the effects of smoking on the baby. A correct response by Anita would be that with cigarette smoking there is increased risk that the baby will have:

a. a low birth weight.
b. a birth defect.
c. anemia.
d. nicotine withdrawal.

Sue Ellen Jennings, 17 years old, is 20 weeks pregnant. She and her husband, Mark, are expecting their first baby.

(THE FOLLOWING 10 ITEMS RELATE TO THE ABOVE PASSAGE.)

7-6
A
Comp.
Asses.

In taking Sue Ellen's prenatal history, which of the following areas concerning her husband would be especially important for the nurse to assess?

a. occupation
b. drug allergies
c. childhood diseases
d. height and weight

7-7
B
Know.
Analy.

The nurse weighs Sue Ellen and finds that she weighs 212 pounds. The nurse realizes that this weight puts Sue Ellen at an increased risk for:

a. cardiac decompensation.
b. cephalopelvic dysproportion.
c. CNS irritability progressing to convulsions.
d. postpartum infection.

7-8
B
Know.
Analy.

Which of the following vital signs for Sue Ellen would be considered in the abnormal range?

a. pulse 88
b. respirations 26
c. temperature 37.4 degrees C
d. blood pressure 135/86

7-9
B
Know.
Analy.

In performing the physical assessment on Sue Ellen, which of the following findings would necessitate referral for further investigation?

a. spider nevi
b. 2+ ankle edema
c. fundus palpated at the umbilicus
d. odorless, cloudy, mucoid vaginal discharge

7-10
B
Know.
Analy.

Which of the following results of Sue Ellen's prenatal lab tests indicates an alteration from expected normal findings?

a. hemoglobin 12.0 g/dL
b. rubella titer 1:8
c. white blood count 11,000
d. nonreactive VDRL

7-11
A
Appl.
Analy.

Sue Ellen tells the nurse that her last normal menstrual period was February 16th, 1987. The nurse calculates Sue Ellen's expected birthing date to be:

a. November 23rd.
b. September 13th.
c. December 28th.
d. December 31st.

45

7-12
A
Know.
Asses.

Besides using the last menstrual period to determine the length of Sue Ellen's pregnancy, which of the following physical findings would also routinely be used?

a. occurrence of quickening
b. rate of the fetal heartbeat
c. calcification of fetal bones on x-ray
d. amniocentesis results

7-13
B
Appl.
Impl.

In assessing fundal height it is important for the nurse to:

a. place the measuring tape at the top of the pubic arch.
b. have Sue Ellen empty her bladder prior to the examination.
c. be aware that fundal height measurements correlate best with weeks of gestation after 32 weeks of pregnancy.
d. realize that maternal height does not affect the reading.

7-14
A
Appl.
Impl.

The nurse assists the physician in performing a pelvic examination on Sue Ellen. In assisting with the pelvic examination, the nurse:

a. has Sue Ellen empty her bladder before the examination.
b. places Sue Ellen in a comfortable semi-Fowler's position.
c. makes sure that Sue Ellen's buttocks are well back toward the middle of the examining table.
d. instructs Sue Ellen to avoid bearing down as the speculum is inserted into the vagina.

7-15
B
Know.
Asses.

In order to determine the adequacy of Sue Ellen's pelvis for birth, which of the following measurements will the physician make vaginally?

a. true conjugate
b. diagonal conjugate
c. transverse outlet diameter
d. obstetrical conjugate

Jennifer Gavin, 19 years old, is in her first trimester of pregnancy. She is interviewed by the nurse on her first prenatal visit.

(THE FOLLOWING 6 ITEMS RELATE TO THE ABOVE PASSAGE.)

7-16
B
Comp.
Asses.

The nurse makes an initial psychosocial assessment. The main purpose of this assessment is to:

a. identify cultural factors Jennifer feels are important.
b. establish a working relationship with Jennifer.
c. determine risk factors of concern to the nurse.
d. discover the areas in which Jennifer has questions.

7-17
C
Comp.
Analy.

Which of the following findings in the psychosocial assessment indicates an alteration from expected normal findings? Jennifer:

a. identifies at least 3 people with whom she feels very comfortable.
b. asks numerous questions regarding the pregnancy.
c. expresses marked anxiety over the diagnosis of pregnancy.
d. states that her husband has been employed as a cook for 2 years.

7-18
D
Comp.
Analy.

Which of the following findings would be considered normal in the psychosocial assessment for the first trimester of pregnancy?

a. an unlisted telephone number
b. initial prenatal visit made at the end of the second trimester
c. parental disapproval of the marriage
d. initial ambivalence regarding the pregnancy

7-19
B
Know.
Plan.

The primary health care provider determines that Jennifer is 10 weeks pregnant. Her next prenatal visit should be in:

a. 2 months.
b. 1 month.
c. 2 weeks.
d. 1 week.

7-20
D
Appl.
Plan.

On Jennifer's second prenatal visit, the nurse continues the psychosocial assessment. Which of the following questions would be most appropriate for the nurse to ask at this time?

a. "What preparations have you and your husband made at home for the baby?"
b. "Have you enrolled in prenatal classes yet?"
c. "Are you planning to have a medicated or an unmedicated birth?"
d. "What body changes have you noticed since your last visit?"

7-21
D
Know.
Asses.

Prior to leaving the office Jennifer is given a written list of danger signals to report immediately. Which one of the following symptoms would be a normal finding not require immediate notification of the health care provider?

a. gush of fluid from vaginal area.
b. constant vomiting
c. facial edema
d. urinary frequency

Jane Lockwood, 26 years old, is in her second trimester of pregnancy. She and her husband, Leon, are coming to the clinic for the third prenatal visit. The Lockwoods are expecting their first baby.

(THE FOLLOWING 3 ITEMS ARE RELATED TO THE ABOVE PASSAGE.)

7-22
D
Appl.
Asses.

Which of the following would not be a part of the normal physical assessment for the third prenatal visit?

a. fundal height
b. weight gain
c. presence of pedal edema
d. 2+ urinary protein

7-23
B
Appl.
Analy.

During the Lockwood's appointment, the nurse performs a prenatal assessment of parenting. Which of the following comments by the Lockwoods would be considered an indication of positive, prenatal, parental role development?

a. "We shouldn't have to change our routine much after the baby is born."
b. "Could I listen to the baby's heartbeat?"
c. "From the way this baby moves, I'll bet he's going to have a temper just like his father."
d. "I really don't think smoking 3 or 4 cigarettes a day can hurt the baby."

7-24
C
Appl.
Impl.

As the Lockwoods get ready to leave the office, Leon comments to the nurse, "I sometimes find it hard to talk to Jane. She seems to be in another world sometimes." The most appropriate response by the nurse would be:

a. "You must make every effort to maintain open communications."
b. "Are you giving Jane enough attention?"
c. "Expectant fathers often feel this way during this time in the pregnancy."
d. "I wouldn't be concerned about it."

Chapter 8

The Expectant Family: Needs and Care

Instructions: For each of the following multiple-choice questions, select the ONE most appropriate answer.

Dena Nolan, 24 years old, is a primigravida in the first trimester of pregnancy who comes to the clinic for her second prenatal visit.

(THE FOLLOWING 5 ITEMS RELATE TO THE ABOVE PASSAGE.)

8-1
C
Comp.
Impl.

Dena complains of "having to go to the bathroom a lot more these days." The nurse explains that this is a common finding in early pregnancy, but that it can mean problems if the frequency is accompanied by:

a. brownish blotches on her cheeks or forehead.
b. a fine red rash on the lower legs.
c. a sense of urgency.
d. leakage of urine with coughing or sneezing.

8-2
A
Know.
Impl.

Dena also mentions that she has had a stuffy nose for about a week but doesn't really seem to have a cold. The nurse explains that the nasal fullness in pregnancy is caused by increased levels of:

a. estrogen.
b. progesterone.
c. chorionic gonadotropin.
d. relaxin.

8-3
D
Comp.
Impl.

In order to relieve the nasal congestion, the nurse suggests that Dena:

a. ask her physician to prescribe a decongestant.
b. use a commercial nasal spray twice each day.
c. use a hot steam vaporizer during the night.
d. put normal saline drops in her nose 3 or 4 times each day.

8-4
B
Appl.
Impl.

Dena comments, "I know I'm not supposed to take medications while I'm pregnant, but just exactly what is wrong with taking aspirin?" The best reply by the nurse would be:

a. "Aspirin causes congenital heart defects."
b. "Aspirin can cause bleeding problems in the baby."
c. "Aspirin can start preterm labor."
d. "Aspirin causes hypoglycemia in pregnant women."

8-5
A
Comp.
Plan.

In providing anticipatory guidance to Dena regarding discomfort she might expect during the second trimester of pregnancy, the nurse should include mention of:

a. hemorrhoids.
b. nose bleeds.
c. breast tenderness.
d. increased vaginal discharge.

Chris Thomas, 27 years old, is a multipara who is 24 weeks pregnant. She comes to the clinic for a regular prenatal visit.

(THE FOLLOWING 7 ITEMS RELATE TO THE ABOVE PASSAGE.)

8-6
B
Comp.
Impl.

Chris complains that she has had several attacks of heartburn since her last appointment. She tells the nurse that a friend told her to take a little sodium bicarbonate (baking soda) in water after she eats. The nurse comments that sodium bicarbonate is not recommended in pregnancy because it:

a. can lead to hypocalcemia.
b. can cause electrolyte imbalance.
c. will only increase the symptoms of heartburn.
d. destroys certain vitamins necessary for growth and development.

8-7
B
Appl.
Impl.

The nurse suggests that Chris might try to relieve her heartburn by:

a. cutting down on the number of meals she eats.
b. avoiding fried foods in her diet.
c. avoiding eating anything 2 or 3 hours before bedtime.
d. lying down after she eats.

8-8
C
Appl.
Impl.

Chris mentions that her mother had "terrible varicose veins" with her pregnancies. Chris asks the nurse if she will get them too. The most appropriate response by the nurse would be:

a. "Why do you ask?"
b. "You're worried about developing varicose veins?"
c. "That's difficult to answer. Poor circulation is also an important factor in the development of varicose veins."
d. "Since you didn't develop varicose veins with your other pregnancies, you're not likely to develop them with this one."

8-9
B
Appl.
Eval.

Chris demonstrates accurate knowledge of the prevention and treatment of varicose veins if she says she will avoid which of the following?

a. elastic stockings
b. crossing her legs
c. elevating her legs
d. wearing panty hose

8-10
A
Appl.
Eval.

If Chris decides to change her method of exercise, the selection of which of the following activities would indicate she understands how to exercise appropriately in late pregnancy?

a. swimming
b. aerobics
c. playing cards
d. tennis

8-11
A
Appl.
Impl.

While discussing the topic of safety hazards during pregnancy, the nurse instructs Chris to avoid or use caution while:

a. taking hot tub baths.
b. wearing a seat belt across her pelvis.
c. continuing her job as secretary for a local insurance agency.
d. receiving immunizations which are made from live attenuated organisms.

8-12
C
Comp.
Impl.

The nurse tells Chris that she might experience a strong, sharp "catching" pain in her lower abdomen and groin area from time to time. The nurse explains that this sensation is due to:

a. exaggerated Braxton-Hicks contractions.
b. a developing urinary tract infection.
c. stretching of the round ligament.
d. pressure of the fetal head on the pelvic nerves.

Rhonda McLeod, 20 years old, is in the last trimester of pregnancy.

(THE FOLLOWING 4 ITEMS RELATE TO THE ABOVE PASSAGE.)

8-13
D
Appl.
Impl.

Rhonda tells the nurse she has had trouble sleeping the last several nights. After assessing Rhonda's sleeping habits, the nurse recommends that Rhonda:

a. drink a cup of hot chocolate or tea just before going to bed.
b. exercise before going to bed so she will be tired and sleep well.
c. ask her physician to order a sleeping pill for her.
d. use several pillows to support her body in positions of rest.

8-14
A
Comp.
Impl.

Rhonda tells the nurse she has heard that fainting can be a problem in late pregnancy. The nurse responds that one of the best ways to avoid passing out is to recognize the approaching signs of fainting which include which one of the following?

a. a decreased ability to hear
b. seeing spots or flashes of bright light before one's eyes
c. a sudden headache
d. irritability

8-15
A
Appl.
Impl.

The nurse instructs Rhonda that if the signs of fainting appear her first action should be to:

a. slowly sit down.
b. get some fresh air.
c. call the physician.
d. breathe slowly into a paper bag.

8-16   Rhonda comments that she and her husband would like to take a trip together before
C   the baby is born. Which of the following responses by the nurse is the most
Appl.   appropriate?
Impl.

    a.   "Air travel after the second trimester is not advised."
    b.   "You should not plan to go more than 100 miles away."
    c.   "Be sure to stop every 2 hours when traveling by car."
    d.   "Foreign travel should be avoided during pregnancy."

Chapter 9

The Expectant Family: Age-Related Considerations

Instructions: For each of the following multiple-choice questions, select the ONE most appropriate answer.

Helen Brown brings her daughter Lydia, 16 years old, to the prenatal clinic for evaluation. Lydia has not had a period for approximately 4 months and she thinks she might be pregnant.

(THE FOLLOWING 5 ITEMS RELATE TO THE ABOVE PASSAGE.)

9-1
C
Know.
Analy.

Lydia's pregnancy is confirmed. Because of Lydia's age, the nurse understands that Lydia is also at risk for having:

a. a cesarean birth.
b. a sexually transmitted disease.
c. a low birth weight baby.
d. placenta previa.

9-2
C
Know.
Analy.

In reviewing Lydia's prenatal history, the nurse finds that Lydia stated that she had used marijuana. The nurse realizes some studies indicate that infants whose mothers used marijuana in pregnancy tended to:

a. be mentally retarded.
b. have more congenital anomalies.
c. be smaller.
d. suffer withdrawal symptoms after birth.

9-3
C
Appl.
Asses.

At the end of the visit Lydia's mother, Helen, comments, "I just don't know how we're going to break this news to Lydia's father." The most appropriate response by the nurse would be:

a. "The best approach would be to just come right out and tell him."
b. "There's no need to rush into things. Wait a month or two."
c. "How have you thought about approaching the matter?"
d. "Would you like me to call your husband and tell him?"

9-4
D
Appl.
Impl.

Helen asks, "And what about Lydia's boyfriend, Eric? He's the father of this baby. What should I do about him?" Which of the following would be the nurse's best response?

a. "It would be best if Lydia did not see him again."
b. "Usually teenage fathers don't want to have anything to do with the young woman once they know there is a pregnancy."
c. "You need to remind Eric that he is legally obligated to support Lydia and the baby."
d. "He may be a source of emotional support to Lydia during the pregnancy."

9-5
C
Appl.
Asses.

Lydia comes in for her second visit four weeks later. She comments to the nurse, "I've gotten used to the idea of this pregnancy. It will be so fun to have a little baby around the house." The most appropriate reply by the nurse would be:

a. "Babies are not fun. They're a lot of work."
b. "I'm so glad to see you're happy about the baby."
c. "Tell me about how you think your life will be after the baby is born."
d. "How are your parents reacting to the baby?"

Cathy Perez, 37 years old, and her husband Bill, 39 years old, are expecting their first baby. Cathy is 12 weeks pregnant. Both are practicing attorneys.

(THE FOLLOWING 4 ITEMS RELATE TO THE ABOVE PASSAGE.)

9-6
D
Appl.
Plan.

In addition to the usual concerns expressed by pregnant women, the nurse is aware that both Cathy and Bill might also express concerns about:

a. the well-being of their fetus.
b. whether or not they will be good parents.
c. whether or not they will be able to afford having this baby.
d. "fitting-in" in prenatal classes.

9-7
C
Know.
Impl.

At her regular clinic appointment Cathy tells the nurse that she is concerned about the possibility of having a baby with Down syndrome. The nurse responds that the incidence of Down syndrome at 37 would be about:

a. 1 in 1000.
b. 1 in 600.
c. 1 in 200.
d. 1 in 50.

9-8
A
Appl.
Asses.

Cathy and Bill tell the nurse they have been thinking about having an amniocentesis. An appropriate response by the nurse would be:

a. "Tell me what you know about this procedure."
b. "That is a good idea. At your age you're at higher risk for developing problems."
c. "That will save you a lot of worry. You'll know today if your baby is normal or not."
d. "Why don't you think it over for a while? Wait a few months yet to make up your minds."

9-9
B
Appl.
Plan.

The amnionic is done, and 2 weeks later the Perezes are told, on a return clinic appointment, that the results of the test indicate their fetus has Down syndrome. After allowing time for the Perezes to express their feelings about this information, an appropriate action for the nurse would be to:

a. refer the Perezes to a genetic counselor.
b. provide the Perezes with information about Down syndrome.
c. help prepare the Perezes for an elective abortion.
d. assure the Perezes that many children with Down syndrome live nearly normal lives.

Chapter 10

Maternal Nutrition

Instructions: For each of the following multiple-choice questions, select the ONE most appropriate answer.

Robbie Rhodes is attending a prenatal nutrition class. This is her first pregnancy and the nurse assesses a knowledge deficit regarding nutrition in general.

(THE FOLLOWING 4 ITEMS RELATE TO THE ABOVE PASSAGE.)

10-1
A
Know.
Impl.

The nurse informs the class that the ability to achieve good prenatal nutrition is influenced by:

a. a general nutritional status prior to pregnancy.
b. ability to follow a written diet.
c. the woman's will power.
d. the success with which the woman adjusts to the pregnancy.

10-2
A
Know.
Asses.

Growth of fetal and maternal tissue requires increased quantities of essential dietary components. The recommended increase for protein during pregnancy for the 23- to 40-year-old age group is:

a. 68%.
b. 33%.
c. 25%.
d. 17%.

10-3
C
Appl.
Impl.

Robbie states, "I have heard that a pregnant woman needs more iron. Is that true?" The nurse's best response would be:

a. "Yes, the pregnant woman, age 23 to 40, needs 100% more iron."
b. "Yes, but the increase is so small the pregnant woman can meet the increased need by eating a well-balanced diet."
c. "Yes, the pregnant woman needs over 250% more iron."
d. "Only pregnant adolescents have an increased need for iron."

10-4
B
Appl.
Impl.

Robbie states, "I am concerned about eating the proper foods during my pregnancy. I am especially concerned about the milk group since I don't really like to drink milk." Which of the following foods should the nurse recommend to her?

a. cottage cheese, dry cereal, 4 oz orange juice
b. cheese, yogurt, custard pudding
c. ice cream, eggs, hot cakes
d. powdered milk, artificial cheese, peanut butter

Wanda King has just had her first pregnancy confirmed. She is 28 years old and has been married for five years. She appears excited and has numerous questions.

(THE FOLLOWING 6 ITEMS RELATE TO THE ABOVE PASSAGE.)

10-5
D
Comp.
Impl.

Wanda is particularly concerned about weight gain. The nurse informs her that optimal weight gain for a pregnant woman depends on her:

a. height.
b. bone structure.
c. prepregnant nutritional state.
d. all of these.

10-6
C
Comp.
Impl.

The nurse explains to Wanda that maternal weight gain should average:

a. 10 to 15 lbs.
b. 16 to 20 lbs.
c. 25 to 30 lbs.
d. 30 to 35 lbs.

10-7
A
Know.
Analy.

A weight gain of _____ during the first trimester of pregnancy is considered ideal.

a. 2 to 4.4 lbs
b. 4.5 to 6 lbs
c. less than 1 lb per week
d. less than 2 lbs

10-8
D
Know.
Analy.

A weight gain of _____ during the last 2 trimesters of pregnancy is considered ideal.

a. slightly more than 4 lbs per week
b. slightly less than 2 lbs per week
c. slightly more than 3 lbs per week
d. slightly less than 1 lb per week

10-9
A
Appl.
Analy.

Wanda visits the clinic during the eleventh week of pregnancy. She has gained 4 pounds above her prepregnant weight. How would the nurse best interpret this data?

a. This weight gain is appropriate and Wanda should be commended for her eating pattern.
b. This small weight gain puts her at risk for intrauterine growth retardation.
c. This large weight gain puts her at risk for preeclampsia.
d. Observation of weight trends for several months is needed to assess adequate weight gains.

10-10
D
Appl.
Analy.

Wanda has gained 5 pounds since her last clinic visit one week ago. How would the nurse interpret this data?

a. This is a normal weight gain during pregnancy.
b. The nurse realizes the need for the same nurse to weigh Wanda weekly to promote consistency.
c. The nurse realizes this inadequate weight gain has been associated with low birth weight.
d. The nurse realizes that this sudden, sharp increase in weight could result from fluid retention and may indicate preeclampsia.

10-11
A
Comp.
Analy.

Women who are 10% or more below their recommended weight prior to conception:

a. have an increased risk of delivering a low birth weight infant and may have an increased risk of developing preeclampsia.
b. have an increased probability of remaining at an optimal weight throughout the entire pregnancy.
c. have an increased risk of anemia which results in a decreased blood volume for the infant.
d. have an increased risk of calcium depletion during pregnancy.

Randy and Janet Kramer explain to the nurse that they are not aware of the type and amount of food Janet should eat during her pregnancy. Janet is 16 weeks pregnant, moderately active, and weighs 132 pounds.

(THE FOLLOWING 7 ITEMS RELATE TO THE ABOVE PASSAGE.)

10-12
B
Appl.
Analy.

In her second trimester Janet will need approximately _____ calories per day.

a. 1800
b. 2400
c. 2800
d. 3400

10-13
B
Comp.
Impl.

Janet asks, "Why is protein so important during pregnancy?" The nurse explains, "Protein is necessary for:

a. development of fetal teeth and bones."
b. blood volume expansion."
c. the development of the fetal nervous system."
d. blood coagulation."

10-14
C
Appl.
Impl.

The nurse informs Janet that all of the following are good sources of protein EXCEPT:

a. chicken, tuna, and rice.
b. fish, spaghetti with meat sauce, and cereal with milk.
c. carrots, peas, and enriched bread.
d. eggs, pork chops, macaroni and cheese, and peanut butter.

10-15
C
Comp.
Asses.

A dietary assessment that indicates Janet is eating a good source of carbohydrates would include which of the following foods?

a. chicken, tuna, and eggs
b. liver, ham, and tomatoes
c. apples, corn, and bread
d. white beans, catfish, and macaroni and cheese

10-16
A
Appl.
Analy.

Janet's blood work demonstrates the following results: Blood type AB positive; hemoglobin 14g; hematocrit 36%; serology nonreactive. How would the nurse best interpret this data?

a. The hematocrit value represents physiologic anemia.
b. Randy will need to be checked for the Rh factor.
c. The baby could acquire congenital syphilis.
d. The baby will develop an ABO incompatibility.

10-17
D
Appl.
Impl.

Janet states, "I don't understand why I have to begin iron supplements since I haven't been taking them thus far during the pregnancy." Which response by the nurse would be most appropriate?

a. "You should have been taking the iron supplements since your first visit. It was an oversight on my part."
b. "Iron supplements are not given during the first trimester because of increased risk of causing preeclampsia."
c. "Iron supplements may not be given during the first trimester because the woman has adequate iron stores and because iron may increase the woman's fluid retention."
d. "Iron supplements may not be given during the first trimester because the increased demand is still minimal and because iron may increase the woman's nausea."

10-18
B
Appl.
Impl.

When counseling Janet concerning foods high in iron, which of the following meals would you recommend to her?

a. tuna sandwich, chocolate pudding, fruit salad
b. chicken liver, tossed salad, dried apricots
c. omelet, raw apple, spinach salad
d. hamburger, french fries, fruit cup

10-19
D
Know.
Analy.

Which of the following could indicate vitamin toxicity?

a. nausea and gastrointestinal upset
b. dryness and cracking of the skin
c. loss of hair
d. all of these

10-20
D
Know.
Analy.

In addition to the knowledge of nutritional needs and food sources, factors that affect a pregnant woman's nutrition include:

a. age.
b. life-style.
c. culture.
d. all of these.

Marion Sanchez, a 14-year-old Mexican American, has just had her pregnancy confirmed. She demonstrates little emotion regarding the pregnancy and does not elaborate when asked questions.

(THE FOLLOWING 5 ITEMS RELATE TO THE ABOVE PASSAGE.)

10-21
A
Appl.
Asses.

During the initial assessment, Marion states that she has been experiencing abdominal distention, generalized discomfort, nausea, loose stools and cramps. These symptoms have existed for years and are recurring in nature. What additional datum should the nurse assess initially? The nurse should:

a. assess the association of these symptoms with milk or food containing milk.
b. assess the association of these symptoms with exercise.
c. evaluate the results from a serum chemical 25 survey.
d. evaluate the results from an abdominal CAT scan.

10-22
D
Comp.
Asses.

From the assessment, the nurse determines that Marion has not reached a gynecological age of 14 years. Which of the following correctly identifies gynecological age?

a. Adolescents who have reached a gynecological age of 14 years are considered physiologically mature.
b. Adolescents who become pregnant at a gynecological age of less than 14 years are at a high biological risk due to their physiological and anatomical immaturity.
c. Nutritional needs are higher for adolescents who have not reached a gynecological age of 14 years.
d. All of these.

10-23
B
Appl.
Impl.

The nurse explains to Marion information specific to adolescent pregnancies. All of the following statements are CORRECT EXCEPT:

a. Young adolescents (13 to 15 years of age) need to gain more weight than older adolescents (16 years of age or older).
b. Intake of as many as 30 calories per kilogram body weight may be needed for young, growing teens who are very active physically.
c. Major factors that determine calorie needs include the amount of physical activity and whether or not the adolescent's growth has been completed.
d. A higher protein intake is recommended for young adolescents.

10-24
A
Appl.
Plan.

Nutritional counseling is an important aspect of Marion's nursing care. Guidance in diet planning for the young adolescent differs from that for an adult. Identify the correct information that should be included in the counseling.

a. Inadequate iron intake is a main concern of the adolescent diet.
b. Excessive intake of calcium is frequently a problem for the pregnant adolescent.
c. Adolescents traditionally eat just three meals a day.
d. RDA for a pregnant teenager and an adult are the same.

10-25
B
Appl.
Impl.

Nutritional counseling interventions for Marion should include all of the following EXCEPT:

a. support individuals, such as the mother, if they will be involved in the food preparation.
b. a negative consequence for inappropriate eating behaviors.
c. the use of present, concrete approaches instead of long-term planning.
d. a group approach.

10-26
C
Comp.
Plan.

A postpartum nutrition plan should consider all of the following EXCEPT:

a. nutritional requirements depend on whether or not the mother decides
   to breast-feed.
b. there is an approximate 10 to 12 pound weight loss after birth.
c. weight loss is most rapid several months after birth.
d. hemoglobin and erythrocyte values should return to normal within 2 to 6 weeks
   postpartum.

10-27
B
Appl.
Impl.

An appropriate intervention for the diagnosis "Alteration in nutrition related to nausea and vomiting" includes:

a. suggest foods high in protein and add small servings of carbohydrates.
b. plan 6 to 8 small feedings per day.
c. limit fluids between meals.
d. limit spicy foods to 1 serving per day.

Chapter 11

Preparation for Parenthood

Instructions: For each of the following multiple-choice questions, select the ONE most appropriate answer.

Len and Vicki Long visit the obstetric clinic to discuss preparation for parenthood.

(THE FOLLOWING 6 ITEMS RELATE TO THE ABOVE PASSAGE.)

11-1
D
Know.
Analy.

Which of the following affect the Long's attitudes, feelings, and fears about parenthood?

a. The relationship they had with their parents.
b. Observations of and encounters with other children.
c. Observations of and encounters with other parents.
d. All of these.

11-2
D
Comp.
Plan.

The nurse's objectives for discussion with the Longs should initially focus on:

a. correcting misconceptions.
b. altering their attitudes and values.
c. calming their fears regarding pregnancy.
d. establishing a caring rapport.

11-3
A
Appl.
Impl.

Vicki states that other parents have told her that many decisions are required when one is preparing for parenthood. The most appropriate nursing response would be:

a. "You will need to decide issues such as type of childbirth preparation, place of birth, choice of the care provider, and activities during the birth."
b. "There are some decisions you will need to make; however, you can avoid several decisions by taking a passive role during the antepartal and intrapartal periods."
c. "Many decisions, such as activities during childbirth and type of childbirth preparation, are made by your care provider. You will need to make decisions such as place of birth and choice of care provider."
d. "You should not worry about the decisions. You will enjoy making them because you will be in control of the situation."

11-4
A
Appl.
Asses.

The nurse's assessment of Len and Vicki, regarding the couple's preparation for parenthood, should include:

a. the couple's information base.
b. the reason they want a drug-free labor.
c. how they compare with other couples.
d. their parents' birth experiences.

11-5
C
Appl.
Plan.

After the nurse completes her assessments of the couple, the appropriate nursing diagnosis is, "Knowledge deficit associated with informational and care needs during pregnancy and childbirth." An appropriate plan should include:

a. identifying learning goals for the couple.
b. making appropriate decisions for the couple.
c. clarifying learning needs and factors that may affect the couples' learning process.
d. telling the couple to establish their goals for childbirth.

11-6
B
Know.
Analy.

The nurse's goal in health teaching for the Longs is to assist them in establishing:

a. compliance with the obstetrician's directions.
b. an information base for self-care practices.
c. a healthful plan to guarantee successful pregnancy outcome.
d. a health plan that they alone direct.

Cameron and Suzanna Dooley are expecting their first baby. Suzanna is one month pregnant and comes to the prenatal clinic for the first time.

(THE FOLLOWING 4 ITEMS RELATE TO THE ABOVE PASSAGE.)

11-7
A
Know.
Plan.

The nurse suggests that Suzanna devise a birth plan. What should be included in this plan?

a. the identification of aspects of the childbearing experience that are most important to the couple
b. only the items/activities that are nonnegotiable
c. activities the couple have done to prepare themselves for childbirth
d. a statement indicating they accept responsibility if the birth plan doesn't work

11-8
A
Comp.
Eval.

What actions taken by Suzanna would indicate appropriate use of the birth plan? Suzanna:

a. shares the birth plan with the care provider and brings it to the birth setting.
b. understands how to develop the birth plan.
c. recognizes that the birth plan is to be shared with the nurse rather than the care provider.
d. sends the plan to the care provider and waits for it to be brought up in conversation.

11-9
D
Appl.
Plan.

Which of the following would the nurse most likely include in the teaching plan for Suzanna? The nurse should include:

a. the educational preparation and skill level of nurse midwives, obstetricians, family practitioners, and lay midwives.
b. information regarding different types of birth settings.
c. means of obtaining further information.
d. all of these.

11-10
C
Appl.
Impl.

Suzanna asks the nurse what choices are available regarding birthing settings. Which of the following is NOT an appropriate nursing response?

a. "The traditional hospital setting, with separate rooms for labor, birth, and postpartal recovery, is an option."
b. "A new type of hospital setting based on family-centered care is now available."
c. "The decision to have the father deliver the baby at home is an option with an uncomplicated pregnancy."
d. "Free-standing birthing centers are very popular."

11-11
A
Appl.
Asses.

As the Daytons seek additional information from couples who have recently given birth, which of the following questions would be appropriate to gather additional information regarding birthing centers?

a. "Was your labor partner/coach treated well?"
b. "Were your labor and birth successful?"
c. "What medications did you take?"
d. "How long was your labor?"

Jim and Karen Grey have been married for 7 years and have 2 children. Their son is 6 years old and their daughter is 5 years old. Karen is 6 months pregnant, and the couple must make a decision about including the children in the birth experience.

(THE FOLLOWING 2 ITEMS RELATE TO THE ABOVE PASSAGE.)

11-12
B
Comp.
Plan.

Which of the following would be appropriate for the nurse to include in the Grey's teaching plan?

a. The decision to have children present at the birth should be made by the physician rather than the parents.
b. Children who will attend a birth should be prepared through books, audiovisual materials, models, and parental discussion.
c. Recent studies have demonstrated a slight increase in bacterial colonization rates in newborns when siblings are present.
d. all of these.

11-13
B
Appl.
Impl.

The decision has been made to have the Grey children present at the birth of the third child. An appropriate nursing intervention at the time of birth would be:

a. suggesting that the children stand at the foot of the bed for a better view.
b. allowing the children to relate to the birth in whatever manner they choose as long as it is not disruptive.
c. informing the children that they must stay in the room until the birth is over.
d. dressing the children in masks and gowns.

11-14
D
Know.
Analy.

Components of the teaching process include:

a. identifying an instructional goal and behavioral objectives.
b. analyzing the characteristics of the learner and the information that needs to be learned.
c. selecting teaching strategies and evaluating of the teaching session.
d. all of these.

11-15 One of the most appropriate ways to assess a group's members' needs is to:
A
Appl.   a. help the group set an agenda.
Asses.   b. evaluate the discussion.
         c. revise the teaching plan.
         d. utilize various teaching methods.

11-16 The nurse is planning a first trimester prenatal class. Which of the following would
B   be appropriate content? The nurse should include:
Comp.
Plan.   a. infant care and feeding.
         b. fetal development and sexuality in pregnancy.
         c. medications and fetal monitoring.
         d. safety issues regarding the newborn.

11-17 The nurse realizes that it is important to include information regarding preparation for
B   cesarean birth because 1 out of every _____ births is cesarean.
Comp.
Analy.   a. 3
         b. 5
         c. 25
         d. 50

11-18 Regardless of the method of childbirth preparation the nurse is teaching, similarities
C   include all of the following EXCEPT:
Comp.
Analy.   a. content to eliminate fear.
         b. relaxation techniques.
         c. the theory of the method chosen.
         d. exercises to condition muscles and breathing patterns used in labor.

11-19 The purpose of relaxation during labor is to:
A
Appl.   a. allow the woman to conserve energy and allow the uterine muscles to work
Analy.   more efficiently.
         b. promote resting and control.
         c. replace unfavorable behaviors with controlled favorable responses.
         d. provide a quiet birth environment.

11-20 When should the woman in labor change from first level breathing to second level
B   breathing? Second level breathing should start:
Appl.
Asses.   a. approximately 1 hour into the labor process.
         b. when level one breathing is no longer effective.
         c. during stage II of labor.
         d. just prior to the actual birth of the child.

11-21   An appropriate nursing intervention related to breathing techniques includes:
A

Appl.   a. telling the woman to place her tongue up behind the front top teeth during
Impl.   breathing to prevent dryness of the mouth.
        b. telling the woman to increase her respiratory rate if she complains of tingling
            in her fingers and/or toes.
        c. telling the woman to pant once active labor begins.
        d. giving the woman a written guide about breathing to read during contractions.

Chapter 12

Pregnancy at Risk

Instructions: For each of the following multiple-choice questions, select the ONE most appropriate answer.

Cindy Bradley, 21 years old, is 12 weeks pregnant with her first baby. Cindy has cardiac disease, class III, as a result of having had childhood rheumatic fever.

(THE FOLLOWING 5 ITEMS RELATE TO THE ABOVE PASSAGE.)

12-1
D
Appl.
Eval.

During a prenatal visit the nurse reviews the signs of cardiac decompensation with Cindy. Cindy demonstrates her understanding of these signs and symptoms if she states that she would notify the physician if which of the following symptoms appeared?

a. an increase in her pulse rate of 10 beats per minute
b. breast tenderness
c. ankle edema
d. a frequent cough

12-2
C
Comp.
Asses.

Signs of cardiac decompensation would be especially likely to appear at:

a. 12 to 16 weeks' gestation.
b. 20 to 24 weeks' gestation.
c. 28 to 32 weeks' gestation.
d. 36 to 40 weeks' gestation.

12-3
B
Comp.
Analy.

In reviewing Cindy's lab results from her initial prenatal visit, which result would alert the nurse to potential problems?

a. urine specific gravity of 1.020
b. hemoglobin of 10 g/dL
c. rubella titer of 1:16
d. total bilirubin of 0.7 mg/dL

12-4
B
Know.
Impl.

Cindy states that she had been taking coumarin but the physician changed her to heparin. She asks the nurse why this was done. The nurse's best response would be:

a. "Heparin may be given by mouth while coumarin must be injected."
b. "Coumarin may cause birth defects in the fetus."
c. "They are the same drug but heparin is less expensive."
d. "Coumarin interferes with iron absorption in the intestines."

12-5 A PRIORITY for Cindy during her pregnancy would be:
A
Appl. a. getting adequate rest.
Plan. b. taking childbirth education classes.
       c. restricting travel.
       d. receiving an influenza immunization.

Rose Terrill, 19 years old, is expecting her first baby. During the history taking, Rose reports that she has been sexually active for 3 years. Two years ago she had gonorrhea which progressed to pelvic inflammatory disease (PID). Prenatal lab tests show that Rose's hemoglobin value is 11.5 g/dL.

(THE FOLLOWING 2 ITEMS RELATE TO THE ABOVE PASSAGE.)

12-6 The nurse notes that Rose's history indicates Rose is at risk for an ectopic pregnancy.
D   Which item from the history below identifies this risk?
Appl.
Analy. a. anemia
       b. sexual activity since age 17
       c. gonorrhea
       d. PID

12-7 In order to determine if Rose has an ectopic pregnancy, the nurse would expect
C   which of the following procedures to be performed?
Appl.
Plan. a. hemoglobin and hematocrit
       b. hCG titer
       c. pelvic examination
       d. amniocentesis

Alberta Napoli, 23 years old, is gravida 4, para 0. At 15 weeks' gestation she is admitted to the maternity unit for a cerclage (Shirodkar-Barter procedure).

(THE FOLLOWING 2 ITEMS RELATE TO THE ABOVE PASSAGE.)

12-8 The purpose of the cerclage is to:
C
Know. a. insure patency of the birth canal.
Analy. b. reattach the placenta.
       c. reinforce a weak cervix.
       d. repair the amniotic sac.

12-9 Alberta has been appropriately prepared for discharge if she comments to the nurse:
B
Appl. a. "I need to avoid intercourse for the duration of my pregnancy."
Eval. b. "I need to come to the hospital at the first sign of labor."
       c. "I realize this will be my last pregnancy."
       d. "I may notice an episode of small to moderate vaginal bleeding during the first
          week I'm home."

67

Jane Russell, 20 years old, is at 16 weeks' gestation. She is admitted to the maternity unit with vaginal bleeding and complains of having moderately heavy, brownish vaginal flow. A diagnosis of complete hydatidiform mole is made using ultrasonography.

(THE FOLLOWING 2 ITEMS RELATE TO THE ABOVE PASSAGE.)

12-10
D
Appl.
Asses.

A priority nursing assessment for Jane would be:

a. fetal heart tones.
b. temperature.
c. urinary output.
d. prolonged bleeding from venipuncture sites.

12-11
A
Appl.
Plan.

The molar pregnancy is evacuated and Jane is prepared for discharge. An essential part of Jane's follow-up care is that she should:

a. not become pregnant for at least one year.
b. receive RhoGAM with the next pregnancy and birth.
c. have her blood pressure checked on a weekly basis for the next 30 days.
d. seek genetic counseling with her partner before the next pregnancy.

Barbara Johnson, 24 years old, is gravida 3, para 0. Barbara comes to the clinic for her initial prenatal visit.

(THE FOLLOWING 3 ITEMS RELATE TO THE ABOVE PASSAGE.)

12-12
B
Comp.
Impl.

During the visit Barbara comments, "My blood type is O negative. Will that cause problems with my pregnancy?" The nurse's best response would be:

a. "There is little likelihood of problems since you are Type O."
b. "What blood type does the baby's father have?"
c. "Have you had problems with your other pregnancies?"
d. "Usually women who have Rh positive blood have problems in pregnancy, not Rh negative women."

12-13
C
Comp.
Asses.

A screening test done to determine if Barbara has been sensitized to the Rh factor is the:

a. L/S ratio.
b. direct Coombs' test.
c. indirect Coombs' test.
d. maternal bilirubin level.

12-14
B
Comp.
Analy.

Following the birth of her Rh positive baby girl, Barbara receives anti-Rh (D) gamma globulin (RhoGAM). The purpose of this medication is to:

a. stimulate Rh sensitization.
b. prevent maternal antibody formation.
c. prevent hemolytic disease in Barbara.
d. convert Barbara's blood to Rh positive.

12-15 Kimberly Sweet, 22 years old, is expecting her second baby in two weeks.
B   Kimberly's blood type is O positive. The nurse might expect blood incompatibility
Know. problems if Kimberly's fetus is:
Plan

    a. Rh negative.
    b. type A.
    c. type O negative.
    d. blood incompatibility problems are highly unlikely in this case.

Sherri Long, 24 years old, is at 30 weeks' gestation. She is admitted to the
emergency room accompanied by her husband Curt. Sherri has an open fracture
of the right radius and ulna. There are several large bruises on her arms, legs, and
abdomen. Curt tells the attending physician that his wife "lost her balance and fell
down a flight of stairs."

(THE FOLLOWING 2 ITEMS RELATE TO THE ABOVE PASSAGE.)

12-16 In addition to assessing Sherri's vital signs, the emergency room nurse should also:
A
Appl.   a. perform a nitrazine test on any vaginal fluid.
Asses.   b. determine urinary protein levels with a dipstick.
    c. check deep tendon reflexes.
    d. assess fetal position using Leopold's maneuvers.

12-17 Surgery is scheduled for open reduction of Sherri's fractured arm. Since Sherri
A   is pregnant, her postoperative nursing care will include:
Appl.
Impl.   a. maintaining Sherri in a side-lying position.
    b. using minimal narcotics to reduce teratogenic effects.
    c. administering oxygen for 24 hours following surgery.
    d. ambulating Sherri within 2 hours after surgery.

Gloria LeBlock, 20 years old, is at 28 weeks' gestation. She comes to the women's
clinic with complaints of a yellowish vaginal discharge and burning on urination.
The prenatal history indicates that Gloria has been sexually active since age 15 and
has had multiple sexual partners.

(THE FOLLOWING 5 ITEMS RELATE TO THE ABOVE PASSAGE.)

12-18 Gloria's vaginal infection is diagnosed as gonorrhea. In teaching Gloria about this
D   disease and its treatment, the nurse's best response would be:
Appl.
Impl.   a. "Because of this infection, your baby will have to be born by cesarean birth."
    b. "You may want to consider a therapeutic abortion."
    c. "You will need to report to the county health department for follow-up care and
       disclosure of your sexual partners."
    d. "No immunity is developed after having gonorrhea."

12-19 Gloria's treatment for gonorrhea will include the administration of:
B
Know.   a. metronidazol (Flagyl.)
Impl.   b. spectinomycin.
    c. podophyllum.
    d. acyclovir (Zovirax).

69

12-20
D
Comp.
Analy.

Gloria's history shows past abuse of drugs including heroin. Urine screening indicates that Gloria has recently used heroin. Drug abuse and addiction puts Gloria at greater risk for:

a. erythroblastosis fetalis.
b. diabetes mellitus.
c. placenta previa.
d. pregnancy-induced hypertension.

12-21
B
Know.
Analy.

The fetus of a heroin-addicted mother, like Gloria, is likely to:

a. be larger for gestational age.
b. have meconium aspiration syndrome.
c. be psychologically addicted to heroin.
d. be postmature due to drug-induced relaxation of muscles.

12-22
A
Know.
Asses.

Because of her history of heroin addiction, Gloria is also screened for:

a. AIDS.
b. syphilis.
c. asymptomatic bacteremia.
d. tuberculosis.

Juanita Redbird, 21 years old, is at 10 weeks' gestation. Her initial prenatal laboratory screening test for rubella showed an antibody titer of less than 1:8.

(THE FOLLOWING 3 ITEMS RELATE TO THE ABOVE PASSAGE.)

12-23
C
Appl.
Impl.

Juanita calls the clinic and tells the nurse that she has been exposed to measles by her sister's little girl. The nurse's best response would be:

a. "Since you are in your first trimester of pregnancy, there is nothing to worry about."
b. "You may want to consider terminating your pregnancy."
c. "Come to the clinic for further evaluation."
d. "You need to receive a rubella vaccination immediately."

12-24
A
Know.
Analy.

A fetus who has been affected by the rubella virus may have:

a. permanent hearing loss.
b. spina bifida.
c. hyperbilirubinemia.
d. phocomelia.

12-25
D
Appl.
Impl.

Laboratory tests indicate that Juanita has had a recent infection with the rubella virus. Upon medical advice, Juanita decides to have a therapeutic abortion. The nurse's best initial comment to Juanita should be:

a. "It's for the best. The baby would no doubt have had many congenital anomalies."
b. "After the abortion you should try to get pregnant as soon as possible."
c. "Would you like me to schedule you with another physician to get a second opinion?"
d. "I realize this has been a difficult decision."

70

12-26   Which of the following is TRUE regarding the cytomegalovirus?
B   Cytomegalovirus:
Know.
Analy.   a. is transmitted through contact with infected cat feces.
          b. can be passed transplacentally to the fetus.
          c. is the least prevalent of the TORCH group of infections.
          d. can be prevented through appropriate vaccination procedures.

Chapter 13

Assessment of Fetal Well-Being

Instructions: For each of the following multiple-choice questions, select the ONE most appropriate answer.

LaWanda Turner, 23 years old, comes to the prenatal clinic after missing one menstrual period. LaWanda has a history of pelvic inflammatory disease (PID).

(THE FOLLOWING 5 ITEMS REFER TO THE ABOVE PASSAGE.)

13-1
D
Appl.
Eval.

The diagnosis of pregnancy is confirmed. Because of LaWanda's history, the physician orders a sonogram. Later the nurse asks whether LaWanda understands why the ultrasound is being done. A response showing LaWanda's understanding would be:

a. "To see if I'm carrying twins."
b. "To see how big the baby is at this point."
c "To see if I'm going to have a boy or a girl."
d. "To see where the baby is growing."

13-2
B
Know.
Asses.

Ultrasound can be used to detect a pregnancy as early as _____ weeks' gestation.

a. 1
b. 6
c. 8
d. 12

13-3
D
Comp.
Impl.

The nurse explains that one of the advantages of ultrasound is that it:

a. causes minimal pain.
b. is considered a noninvasive procedure.
c. provides test results within one week.
d. does not use ionizing radiation.

13-4
A
Know.
Asses

When using ultrasound to determine fetal age, which fetal measurement is most widely used?

a. biparietal diameter of the fetal head
b. crown-rump length
c. total fetal length
d. head-to-abdomen ratio

13-5
C
Appl.
Impl.

In assisting with the ultrasound, the nurse:

a. obtains informed consent from LaWanda prior to the procedure.
b. has LaWanda empty her bladder before the test begins.
c. assists LaWanda into a supine position on the examining table.
d. instructs LaWanda to eat a fat-free meal 2 hours before the scheduled test time.

Sally Ratcliff, 26 years old, is at 28 weeks' gestation. Her fundal height measurement at this clinic appointment is 25 centimeters.

(THE FOLLOWING 6 ITEMS RELATE TO THE ABOVE PASSAGE.)

13-6
B
Appl.
Impl.

A sonogram is ordered by Sally's health care provider. The nurse tells Sally that the main purpose of this test is to:

a. assess for congenital anomalies.
b. evaluate fetal growth.
c. grade the placenta.
d. rule out a suspected hydatidiform mole.

13-7
B
Comp.
Analy.

In addition to the ultrasound test, a nonstress test is also performed to complete a biophysical profile for Sally's fetus. A score for the profile which would indicate the fetus is normal would be:

a. over 10.
b. 8 to 10.
c. 3 to 7.
d. 0 to 2.

13-8
D
Appl.
Impl.

Sally is asked to keep a fetal activity diary and bring the results with her to her next clinic visit. One week later she calls the clinic and anxiously tells the nurse that she has not felt the baby move for over 30 minutes. The most appropriate initial comment by the nurse would be:

a. "You need to come to the clinic right away for further evaluation."
b. "Have you been smoking?"
c. "When did you eat last?"
d. "Your baby may be asleep."

13-9
A
Appl.
Eval.

At 32 weeks' gestation, Sally is scheduled for another nonstress test. The nurse asks Sally if she remembers how to prepare for the test. An appropriate response by Sally would be:

a. "I have to lie still during the test."
b. "I'll have an IV started before the test."
c. "I must avoid drinks containing caffeine 24 hours before the test."
d. "I need to have a full bladder."

13-10
C
Appl.
Asses.

During the nonstress test the nurse notes that fetal heart rate decelerates about 15 beats during a period of fetal movement. The decelerations occur twice during the test and last 20 seconds each. The nurse realizes these results will be interpreted as:

a. a negative test.
b. a reactive test.
c. a nonreactive test.
d. an unsatisfactory test.

13-11
C
Appl.
Plan.

Based on the nonstress test results, the nurse would prepare Sally for:

a. a return appointment for an ultrasound examination in 2 weeks.
b. a return appointment in 1 week for a repeat nonstress test.
c. a contraction stress test.
d. hospitalization with fetal monitoring.

Kay Richards, 27 years old, has had chronic hypertension for 3 years. She is 33 weeks pregnant and comes to the high-risk screening center for a contraction stress test.

(THE FOLLOWING 4 ITEMS RELATE TO THE ABOVE PASSAGE.)

13-12
B
Comp.
Analy.

The nurse understands that the contraction stress test is being performed in order to determine:

a. what effect Kay's hypertension has had on the fetus.
b. if the placental reserve is adequate for labor.
c. if fetal movement increases with contractions.
d. what effect contractions will have on Kay's blood pressure.

13-13
D
Comp.
Analy.

Hyperstimulation during the nipple stimulation test occurs when:

a. the fetal heart rate decelerates when 3 contractions occur within a 10-minute period.
b. the fetal heart rate accelerates when contractions last up to 60 seconds.
c. there are more than 5 fetal movements in a 10-minute period.
d. the fetal heart rate decelerates when contractions last more than 90 seconds.

13-14
D
Appl.
Analy.

During the oxytocin challenge test, the nurse notes that the test is positive if Kay has:

a. no decelerations with 3 contractions in 10 minutes.
b. accelerations of the fetal heart rate with fetal movement.
c. contractions lasting longer than 90 seconds.
d. late decelerations with more than 50% of the contractions.

13-15
D
Appl.
Analy.

The nurse realizes that a positive oxytocin challenge test for Kay means that:

a. Kay will need to have the oxytocin challenge test repeated in about one week.
b. more pain medication will be required when Kay does go into labor.
c. the use of oxytocin causes Kay's blood pressure to become elevated.
d. Kay may have to have a cesarean birth.

Collette Fisher, 28 years old, has been an insulin-dependent diabetic for 10 years. She is 34 weeks pregnant and comes for her appointment at the high-risk prenatal clinic.

(THE FOLLOWING 9 ITEMS REFER TO THE ABOVE PASSAGE.)

13-16
B
Appl.
Impl.
Collette's pregnancy will be monitored by urinary estriol levels. The nurse's explanation of this test should include which of the following?

  a. "Bring in a sample of the first morning voiding in a clean container to your next clinic appointment."
  b. "Be sure you collect all of your urine in a 24-hour period."
  c. "Results of this test will take about 5 days to determine."
  d. "You may be asked to do another 24-hour collection in another week."

13-17
B
Comp.
Analy.
An abnormal finding for a serial 24-hour urinary estriol test would be:

  a. a steady increase in estriol levels over the series of collection.
  b. a value of 10 mg/24 hours.
  c. a value of 32 mg/24 hours.
  d. a drop of 10% below the preceding estriol test.

13-18
C
Appl.
Eval.
Two weeks later Collette is scheduled for an amniocentesis. She demonstrates understanding of the purpose for the test by stating, "The amniocentesis is done to see if:

  a. the baby has Down syndrome."
  b. the baby is a boy or a girl."
  c. the baby is mature enough to be born."
  d. I have an intrauterine infection."

13-19
A
Appl.
Eval.
The nurse asks Collette to explain what the health care provider told her about the risks of this procedure. Collette correctly responds:

  a. "I might go into labor early."
  b. "It could produce a congenital defect in my baby."
  c. "Actually, there are no real risks to this procedure."
  d. "The test could stunt my baby's growth."

13-20
C
Comp.
Analy.
Just prior to having the amniocentesis, Collette has an ultrasound done. The purpose of an ultrasound at this time is to:

  a. determine if there is more than one fetus.
  b. prescreen the fetus for gross congenital anomalies.
  c. locate the placenta.
  d. estimate the fetal age.

13-21
C
Appl.
Impl.
Collette asks the nurse if the amniocentesis will hurt. The nurse should initially reply by saying:

  a. "There will be very little discomfort."
  b. "You will have an epidural or spinal anesthetic so you won't feel anything."
  c. "There will be some discomfort when the needle is inserted into your abdomen."
  d. "Would you like to talk to other women who have had this procedure?"

13-22   The nurse prepares Collette for the amniocentesis by:
A
Appl.   a. having her empty her bladder.
Impl.   b. starting an intravenous infusion.
         c. administering oxygen with a non-rebreathing face mask.
         d. having her assume a comfortable position on her left side.

13-23   Several tests are performed on the sample of Collette's amniotic fluid. One of
A   these tests is the lecithin/sphingomyelin (L/S) ratio. The ratio for Collette is 2:1.
Comp.   Since she is a diabetic, this result indicates the fetus:
Analy.
         a. may have immature lungs.
         b. has an intrauterine infection.
         c. has a neural tube defect.
         d. is at risk for hyperglycemia.

13-24   A test result on the amniotic fluid which would indicate that the fetus is in no
D   apparent distress at this time would be:
Appl.
Analy.   a. a creatinine level of 1.5 mg/dL.
         b. 8% of the fat cells stained orange with Nile blue sulfate.
         c. a mild amount of meconium present.
         d. the absence of bilirubin in the fluid.

PART 3

BIRTH

Chapter 14

Processes and Stages of Birth

Instructions: For each of the following multiple-choice questions, select the ONE most appropriate answer

Jean Price, a 24-year-old primigravida, is admitted to the labor and delivery suite of the hospital. She is accompanied by her husband Tom. The couple tell the nurse that this is the first hospital admission for Jean. They have recently completed the prepared childbirth course sponsored by the hospital.

(THE FOLLOWING 9 ITEMS RELATE TO THE ABOVE PASSAGE.)

14-1
B
Comp.
Asses.

Jean tells the nurse, "I'm not sure this is it. I have had one episode of false labor before." Which of the following clinical manifestations is most indicative of true labor?

a. increased bloody show
b. effacement and dilation of the cervical os
c. sudden burst of energy
d. contraction and relaxation of the uterus

14-2
D
Comp.
Asses.

The nurse continues her assessment of Jean. In order to BEST assess for the duration of the contractions, the nurse should:

a. palpate just above the symphysis pubis.
b. ask Jean about her contractions.
c. observe Jean's behavior and facial expression.
d. palpate the uterine fundus.

14-3
A
Comp.
Analy.

The nurse asks Jean how frequently her contractions have been coming. Jean gives the nurse a paper with the following times: 12:05 a.m., 12:10 a.m., 12:15 a.m., 12:20 a.m. The frequency of Jean's contractions is every:

a. 5 minutes.
b. 10 minutes.
c. 2 minutes.
d. 15 minutes.

14-4
C
Know.
Asses.

The nurse also needs to know the duration of the uterine contractions. The duration of the contraction is measured from the:

a. beginning of one contraction to the beginning of another contraction.
b. end of a contraction to the beginning of the next contraction.
c. beginning of the contraction until the end of the same contraction.
d. end of a contraction to the end of the next contraction.

14-5
D
Appl.
Impl.

Jean states that her contractions feel "pretty strong." The nurse assesses the next three contractions and her fingers are unable to indent the uterine wall. The intensity of this type of contraction would be termed:

a. slight.
b. mild.
c. moderate.
d. strong.

14-6
B
Know.
Asses.

The nurse needs to determine fetal presentation prior to assessing the fetal heart. "Presentation" refers to the:

a. relationship of the presenting part to the pelvis.
b. part of the fetal body entering the pelvis.
c. flexion and extension of the fetal body and extremities.
d. relationships of the cephalocaudal axis of the fetus to the maternal spine.

14-7
C
Know.
Asses.

The nurse reviews the copy of the client's antepartum records sent by her obstetrician's office. The records indicate that Jean's pelvic structure is android. Of the following, the type of maternal pelvis most favorable for a vaginal delivery is:

a. polypoid.
b. android.
c. gynecoid.
d. platypelloid.

14-8
A
Comp.
Impl.

The nurse performs a vaginal examination on Jean and determines that the biparietal diameter of the fetal head has reached the pelvic inlet. The fetus is best described as:

a. engaged.
b. at the level of the ischial spines.
c. floating.
d. at zero station.

14-9
B
Appl.
Impl.

Jean asks the nurse, "Do you think I will have an easy labor?" The best response by the nurse would be:

a. "There is no way to know how your labor will proceed."
b. "There are several interrelated factors that determine the length and difficulty of your labor."
c. "Labor means hard work."
d. "We have lots of pain relief measures if it gets too bad."

14-10
B
Know.
Asses.

The mechanism of labor which allows the smallest anteroposterior diameter of the fetal head to present itself to the maternal pelvis is:

a. descent.
b. flexion.
c. internal rotation.
d. extension.

14-11
C
Know.
Asses.

The most intense portion of the uterine contraction is termed the:

a. increment.
b. decrement.
c. acme.
d. peak.

14-12
D
Know.
Asses.

The hormone that acts to inhibit the development of uterine contractions is:

a. estrogen.
b. oxyotocin.
c. prostaglandin.
d. progesterone.

14-13
D
Comp.
Analy.

The blood pressure of a laboring woman, taken during a contraction, is 30/21 mm Hg over her baseline admission blood pressure of 110/70. The nurse realizes that the uterine contractions of labor will produce a/an:

a. decreased cardiac output leading to decreased blood pressure.
b. increased systolic blood pressure leading to widening pulse pressure.
c. pooling of blood in the intervillous space leading to decreased cardiac output.
d. increased peripheral resistance leading to increased systolic and diastolic blood pressure.

Elena Marquez is a 19-year-old Mexican-American primigravida. She is accompanied to the labor and delivery suite by her 25-year-old husband Jose and her mother-in-law who is from Mexico.

(THE FOLLOWING 5 ITEMS RELATE TO THE ABOVE PASSAGE.)

14-14
D
Comp.
Plan.

In planning care for Elena during the labor and birth process, the nurse recognizes that the MOST relevant consideration is Elena's:

a. past experiences and perception of pain.
b. cultural patterns of behavior about the maternal role in childbirth.
c. type of childbirth preparation.
d. perception of her role during the labor process.

14-15
C
Appl.
Impl.

Elena and Jose have recently completed prepared childbirth classes. They were taught a variety of pain control techniques to use during the labor process. The technique which acts to "close the gate" to painful uterine contractions is:

a. breathing.
b. distraction.
c. cutaneous stimulation.
d. hypnosis.

14-16
D
Comp.
Analy.

In the first state of labor Elena wants to know why she has pain in other places if it is her cervix that is stretching and opening. The nurse understands that the PRIMARY reason for the additional discomfort is:

a. distention of the vagina.
b. pressure of the presenting part on the floor of the perineum.
c. muscle tension in the arms and legs.
d. referred pain from the uterus.

14-17
D
Appl.
Impl.

Elena complains of increasing rectal pressure. A vaginal examination reveals a cervix that is 8 centimeters dilated and 100% effaced. The head is at +2 station. The nurse realizes that:

a. Elena may start to push with the next contraction.
b. Elena should deliver within the next 30 minutes.
c. the baby is very high and she will need to do a lot of pushing.
d. the fetus has descended farther down into the birth canal.

14-18
C
Appl.
Impl.

Elena begins to display signs of irritability and restlessness. She states, "I can't take this anymore." The nurse explains to Elena that her behavior:

a. should it continue, will interfere with this stage of labor.
b. is inappropriate for a married woman of her cultural background.
c. is to be expected at this phase of the labor process.
d. is frightening the other clients and must stop immediately.

14-19
C
Know.
Asses.

The process of taking-up the cervical canal by the uterine walls and changing it into a paper thin circular structure is known as:

a. engagement.
b. labor.
c. effacement.
d. dilation.

14-20
A
Appl.
Impl.

The client observes the vaginal birth of her first child by looking in the mirror in the birthing room. She tells the nurse that after the birth of the baby's head, with the face looking at the floor, the head turned to the right on its own without being touched. The nurse tells the client that this is a normal mechanism called:

a. external rotation.
b. flexion.
c. extension.
d. internal rotation.

14-21
D
Appl.
Impl.

A primigravida client tells the nurse that about 2 weeks before she went into labor she noticed her breathing became easier, but she had to go to the bathroom more frequently. The nurse tells the client that what she experienced is commonly called:

a. quickening.
b. dilation.
c. dropping.
d. lightening.

14-22
D
Appl.
Impl.

A primigravida client asks the labor room nurse why she is still undelivered while the other lady who was admitted after she was has just had her baby. The nurse realizes the other client was a gravida 3, para 3. The nurse's response should be based on the knowledge that the:

a. primigravida came to the hospital too early.
b. multiparous client had better contractions.
c. multiparous client was more experienced in childbirth.
d. primigravida must efface before dilating.

14-23
C
Appl.
Asses.

The laboring client is having contractions every 2 to 3 minutes, lasting 60 to 90 seconds and of strong intensity. The fetal head is visualized when the client pushes involuntarily. A vaginal examination reveals a completely dilated and effaced cervix. The nurse assesses the client to be in what stage of labor?

a. transition
b. third
c. second
d. active

14-24
D
Appl.
Impl.

The client screams at the the nurse to "leave me alone!" The nurse should:

a. ask another nurse to stay with the client.
b. ask the client why she wants the nurse to leave her alone.
c. leave the room immediately.
d. remain with the client.

14-25
C
Appl.
Asses.

The client has delivered a healthy infant and is now being taken to the recovery room. The PRIORITY assessment the nurse must make of the client immediately after birth is for:

a. observation for nausea and vomiting.
b. urinary retention.
c. hemodynamic changes.
d. elevation of temperature.

Chapter 15

Intrapartal Nursing Assessment

Instructions: For each of the following multiple-choice questions, select the ONE most appropriate answer.

Maggie Charles is admitted to the labor and delivery suite in early labor. This is her first baby and first hospitalization. She and her husband, Mike, have completed a prepared childbirth course. While obtaining a client history, the nurse notices that Maggie is continually twisting her wedding band and giggles nervously after answering questions.

(THE FOLLOWING 8 ITEMS RELATE TO THE ABOVE PASSAGE.)

15-1
B
Appl.
Asses.

The nurse asks Maggie if she is anxious about something and Maggie responds by saying, "No." The nurse assesses Maggie's behavior as:

  a. not an accurate indicator of her real feelings.
  b. incongruent with her verbal statement.
  c. habitual mannerism.
  d. inappropriate for the situation.

15-2
D
Comp.
Asses.

Ongoing, critical, intrapartal assessments of Maggie would NOT include:

  a. fetal heart rate.
  b. maternal vital signs.
  c. labor status.
  d. maternal weight.

15-3
B
Know.
Asses.

Maggie tells the nurse that she thinks her water has broken. Which of the following tests is carried out to check for ruptured membranes?

  a. shake test
  b. nitrazine test
  c. dextrostix test
  d. urinalysis

15-4
D
Know.
Asses.

It is determined that Maggie's membranes are intact and the nurse proceeds with the initial intrapartal assessment. The vaginal examination that is performed does NOT reveal information about:

  a. cervical effacement and dilation.
  b. fetal position and presentation.
  c. membrane status.
  d. uterine contraction status.

15-5
A
Know.
Asses.

The nurse determines the fetal presentation by performing Leopold's maneuvers. The second maneuver is used to determine:

a. whether the fetal head or buttocks occupies the uterine fundus.
b. the location of the fetal back.
c. whether the head or buttocks lies in the pelvic inlet.
d. the descent of the presenting part into the pelvis.

15-6
D
Appl.
Plan.

The nurse needs to determine the fetal heart rate (FHR). She has determined that the fetal back is located toward Maggie's left side, the small part toward the right side, and that there is a vertex presentation. The initial quadrant to begin auscultating the heart rate is the:

a. right upper quadrant.
b. right lower quadrant.
c. left upper quadrant.
d. left lower quadrant.

15-7
B
Know.
Asses.

The nurse obtains a FHR of 144 beats per minute (BPM). The normal baseline range for a FHR is:

a. 100 to 160 beats per minute.
b. 120 to 160 beats per minute.
c. 130 to 180 beats per minute.
d. 110 to 150 beats per minute.

15-8
C
Comp.
Plan.

The nurse decides not to initiate external electronic fetal monitoring in this situation. The major disadvantage of utilizing these devices for Maggie would be:

a. inability to detect normal baseline changes.
b. too much distraction from machines and noise.
c. restriction of maternal movement.
d. inability to determine the intensity of uterine contractions.

Maggie has been in the labor suite for approximately one hour. Her husband, Mike, rejoined her once the admission procedures were completed. Since she displayed anxious behavior during admission, the nurse reassesses her present level of anxiety.

(THE FOLLOWING 3 ITEMS RELATE TO THE ABOVE PASSAGE.)

15-9
A
Appl.
Eval.

Maggie is using her breathing techniques effectively during her contractions. Her husband is assisting her and reminding her to stay relaxed. The nurse decides that:

a. Maggie is able to cope at this phase of her labor.
b. she needs to assume a greater role in supporting Maggie.
c. she needs to suggest some alternative coping mechanism to the couple.
d. the couple do not need her presence during labor.

15-10
B
Comp.
Analy.

The nurse notes that the FHR slows from its baseline of 144 BPM to 126 BPM from the acme of the contraction. The FHR then returns to its baseline by the end of the contraction. The nurse understands that this is indicative of:

a. fetal hypoxia.
b. fetal head compression.
c. deterioration of the placental unit.
d. maternal hypoxia.

15-11
D
Appl.
Impl.

Maggie's most recent vaginal examination reveals that she is 10 centimeters dilated and pushing. The nurse should now begin to check the FHR:

a. for a full minute.
b. during each contraction.
c. every 5 minutes.
d. immediately after each contraction.

Angela Mazzio, a 32-year-old gravida 2, comes to the hospital in active labor. She tells the admitting nurse that she is a diabetic. When asked about her previous pregnancy and birth, Angela tells the nurse she delivered a stillborn 2 years before. The nurse immediately initiates indirect fetal heart rate monitoring.

(THE FOLLOWING 13 ITEMS RELATE TO THE ABOVE PASSAGE.)

15-12
A
Comp.
Plan.

The best device to utilize to provide for indirect fetal heart rate monitoring is the:

a. transducer.
b. fetal scalp electrode.
c. fetoscope.
d. ultrasound stethoscope.

15-13
C
Comp.
Plan.

Once the admission procedures are completed, the nurse begins to gather equipment for direct fetal heart rate monitoring. The rationale for using direct monitoring is:

a. direct monitoring can be used throughout the labor process.
b. indirect monitoring is subject to artifacts.
c. the spiral electrode provides more accurate data than external monitoring.
d. fetal distress can be more readily detected.

15-14
D
Know.
Asses.

Angela tells the nurse she thinks her membranes have ruptured. The nurse uses reagent paper to test the fluid. If Angela's membranes are truly ruptured, the reagent paper should turn:

a. red.
b. yellow.
c. green.
d. blue.

84

15-15   Angela's membranes have ruptured. The nurse should:
C
Appl.   a. change the perineal pad.
Impl.   b. call the physician.
         c. check the fetal heart rate (FHR).
         d. position Angela on her right side.

15-16   The nurse sees that the amniotic fluid is meconium stained. Since Angela has a
D   vertex presentation, the nurse should:
Appl.
Impl.   a. change Angela's position.
         b. notify the physician.
         c. administer oxygen.
         d. check the fetal heart rate (FHR).

15-17   The nurse immediately performs a vaginal examination to determine cervical status,
C   to check the internal fetal heart rate monitoring, and, primarily, to assess for:
Comp.
Asses.   a. fetal descent.
         b. fetal position change.
         c. prolapsed umbilical cord.
         d. caput succedaneum.

15-18   The nurse notices that the FHR begins to decline from its baseline of 144 BPM to
C   110 BPM after the acme of each contraction. The wave is uniform with a shape
Appl.   reflecting the contraction. The nurse recognizes this deviation as a/an:
Asses.
         a. fetal bradycardia.
         b. early deceleration.
         c. late deceleration.
         d. variable deceleration.

15-19   The fetal factor which makes electronic fetal monitoring necessary in this situation
C   is:
Know.
Asses.   a. decreased fetal movement.
         b. intrauterine growth retardation.
         c. meconium passage.
         d. postmaturity.

15-20   The nurse documents the previous events on the fetal heart rate tracing. Which of
B   the following data is most accurate and informative?
Appl.
Impl.   a. Amniotomy with clear fluid; vaginal examination.
         b. Spontaneous rupture of membrane (SROM) with meconium-stained fluid;
             vaginal examination results; scalp electrode applied.
         c. SROM; vaginal examination; oxygen administration.
         d. Artificial ROM; scalp electrode applied.

15-21
A
Appl.
Impl.

The nurse's initial response to this alteration in fetal heart rate pattern should be to:

a. turn Angela to her left side.
b. monitor maternal blood pressure.
c. administer oxygen.
d. assess maternal hydration status.

15-22
D
Appl.
Impl.

Angela asks why she needs to have the internal fetal monitoring. The nurse's best intervention would be to:

a. reassure Angela that her baby is fine.
b. refer the question to the physician.
c. tell Angela that release of meconium indicates fetal distress.
d. explain to Angela that she needs to observe the baby more closely.

15-23
A
Know.
Asses.

The physician is notified of the periodic change in the FHR and decides assessment of fetal acid base status is necessary. The blood pH obtained by fetal sampling of a severely depressed fetus would be:

a. 7.1.
b. 7.2.
c. 7.3.
d. 7.4.

15-24
C
Appl.
Plan.

The results of the fetal scalp sampling and the other clinical manifestations lead the physician to diagnose a severely depressed fetus. The appropriate nursing action at this time would be to:

a. increase the oxygen being administered to Angela.
b. change Angela's position again.
c. prepare Angela for a cesarean birth.
d. start an intravenous infusion.

Gloria Perry, a laboring primigravida, has had the external monitoring applied by the nurse. The nurse periodically places her hand on Gloria's fundus during the contractions. Gloria asks if everything is all right.

(THE FOLLOWING 3 ITEMS RELATE TO THE ABOVE PASSAGE.)

15-25
C
Appl.
Impl.

The nurse's best response to explain her behavior to Gloria would be:

a. "I need to make sure that the machine is working properly."
b. "Sometimes the monitors don't give accurate readings."
c. "With this type of monitoring, palpating a few of your contractions gives me a better idea of how strong they really are."
d. "I would rather do this the old-fashioned way."

15-26
D
Comp.
Analy.

The nurse periodically examines the fetal monitor tracing. Gloria asks why this is necessary when the heart rate is normal. Which of the following statements best explains the nurse's behavior?

a. "The fetal heart rate tracing is a legal document that must be checked for accuracy."
b. "Examination of the fetal heart rate tracing can help predict the fetal outcome."
c. "The fetal monitor records data but the nurse must interpret the information."
d. "A fetus that is in distress may have a normal heart rate but demonstrate subtle changes that can indicate a potential problem."

15-27
D
Know.
Asses.

Which of the following is NOT a change in the baseline FHR?

a. tachycardia
b. bradycardia
c. beat-to-beat variability
d. acceleration

Chapter 16

The Family in Childbirth: Needs and Care

Instructions: For each of the following multiple-choice questions, select the ONE most appropriate answer.

Claire Johnson, a 20-year-old primagravida, is brought to the hospital in active labor by her husband,Leland. She is brought by wheelchair to the birthing area and greeted by the nurse.

16-1
C
Comp.
Asses.

What is the nurse's priority in the admission assessment of Claire? S/he must:

a. determine the couple's goals for the birth experience.
b. assess Clair's coping mechanisms.
c. assess the imminence of birth.
d. determine the presence or absence of a support system.

16-2
C
Comp.
Impl.

Claire tells the nurse the contractions are coming about every 20 minutes and last about 30 seconds. Further examination by the nurse gives the following data: FHR 140 BPM; cervix 100% effaced and 3 cm dilated; presenting station -1; membranes intact. According to Friedman's terminology, Claire is in what phase of labor?

a. transition
b. active phase
c. latent phase
d. phase of maximum slope

16-3
B
Appl.
Analy.

The nurse observes Claire during contractions and sees her grimace. Claire says the contractions feel like menstrual cramps and that she is glad to be in labor. The nurse assesses this behavior and statement as:

a. incongruent.
b. being expected during this phase of labor.
c. being inappropriate for a primigravida.
d. being euphoric.

16-4
A
Comp.
Analy.

Having completed her/his initial assessment of Claire, and having determining that birth is not imminent, the nurse begins to plan for care of the laboring couple. Her/his nursing diagnosis at this time would most likely be:

a. potential alteration in comfort.
b. ineffective individual coping.
c. knowledge deficit.
d. anxiety.

16-5
A
Comp.
Plan.

By inquiring about Claire's expectations for her labor and delivery, the nurse is PRIMARILY:

a. recognizing Claire as an active participant in her own care.
b. attempting to correct any misinformation Claire may have received.
c. acting as a patient advocate.
d. promoting the establishment of rapport with Claire.

16-6
D
Know.
Plan.

The physician has a standing order for a cleansing enema. The PRIMARY purpose of administering a cleansing enema during labor is to:

a. stimulate uterine contractions.
b. prevent contamination of the sterile field during birth.
c. facilitate vaginal examinations.
d. evacuate the lower bowel.

16-7
C
Know.
Asses.

During this phase of Claire's labor her fetus' FHR should be assessed every:

a. 15 minutes for 5 seconds.
b. 30 minutes for 15 seconds.
c. hour for 15 minutes.
d. 2 hours for 30 minutes.

16-8
B
Appl.
Plan.

Considering the client's condition and phase in labor, the nurse anticipates that Claire's activity orders will be:

a. complete bed rest.
b. ambulation ad lib.
c. bathroom privileges.
d. up in chair.

16-9
C
Comp.
Plan.

The nurse can best utilize this period of early labor for:

a. teaching Claire about newborn care.
b. dispelling myths about childbirth.
c. teaching breathing techniques for use during labor.
d. allowing Claire to rest as much as possible.

Rena Markowitz is a 24-year-old multipara. During admission, the nurse assesses the contractions are occurring every 3 minutes and lasting 45 seconds. Rena says she has been in labor for approximately 10 hours.

(THE FOLLOWING 9 ITEMS RELATE TO THE ABOVE PASSAGE.)

16-10
B
Comp.
Asses.

The PRIORITY assessment the nurse needs to make at this time is the:

a. time Rena last ate.
b. cervical dilation
c. allergies to medications.
d. oral temperature.

16-11
B
Appl.
Plan.

Rena initially took a prepared childbirth class before the birth of her first child and did not repeat the class with this pregnancy. The nurse should encourage which of the following breathing patterns?

a. cleansing breath; slow, deep chest breathing; cleansing breath
b. cleansing breath; accelerated chest breathing; cleansing breath
c. hee-hee, hee-ho breathing
d. pant-pant, blow breathing

16-12
C
Appl.
Impl.

Rena was unable to reach her husband before coming to the hospital. In this situation the best nursing action would be to:

a. provide her with ice chips for comfort.
b. assist her with position changes.
c. provide support and reassurance.
d. encourage her to void every 1 to 2 hours for comfort.

16-13
D
Appl.
Asses.

Rena tells the nurse her contractions are getting harder and that she is getting tired. She is very anxious and asks the nurse not to leave her alone. Considering Rena's behavior, the nurse assesses her to be dilated how many centimeters?

a. 0 to 2
b. 2 to 3
c. 4 to 7
d. 8 to 10

16-14
C
Comp.
Analy.

During the miniprep and during each of the vaginal examinations, Rena continually tries to pull her hospital gown down to cover her perineum. The nurse understands the client's behavior reflects her:

a. lack of understanding of hospital procedures.
b. attempt to keep warm.
c. attempt to preserve her privacy.
d. noncompliance.

16-15
C
Appl.
Impl.

The nurse rechecks Rena's blood pressure and finds it has dropped. In order to decrease the incidence of supine hypotension, the nurse should encourage Rena to remain in which position?

a. semi-Fowler's
b. supine
c. left lateral
d. tailor-sitting

16-16
A
App.
Impl.

Rena's contractions are every 2 to 3 minutes, lasting 90 seconds, and are very strong. A vaginal examination reveals the client is 9 cm dilated and +2 station. The nurse can best promote comfort during this transition phase by:

a. applying pressure to Rena's sacrum.
b. washing Rena's perineum.
c. encouraging Rena to void.
d. placing a cool cloth behind Rena's neck.

16-17
D
Know.
Asses.

Rena complains of tingling in her fingers and around her mouth. The nurse realizes that these are clinical manifestations of:

a. hypercapnia.
b. anxiety.
c. imminent birth.
d. hyperventilation.

16-18
C
Know.
Impl.

The nurse extends her hand toward the client during a contraction. The nurse knows that which of the following is TRUE regarding the use of touch during the childbirth process? The use of touch during childbirth:

a. is culturally dependent.
b. is dependent upon the individual need of the client.
c. is dependent upon the client's stage of labor.
d. should only be done by the significant other.

16-19
B
Know.
Plan.

The birthing position which is anatomically preferred for ease of birth, as well as for fetal and maternal well-being, is the _____ position.

a. side-lying
b. sitting
c. squatting
d. lithotomy

16-20
C
Appl.
Impl.

The nursing intervention which promotes the nursing goal of parental attachment would be:

a. allowing the mother to rest immediately after birth.
b. transferring the infant to the newborn nursery for its initial assessment.
c. positioning the baby for eye contact with the mother.
d. placing the infant in the warmer.

16-21
B
Know.
Eval.

A client's physician has ordered an oxytocic drug to be given after the birth of an infant. The nurse knows that if this drug is effective the client will have:

a. decreased uterine contractions.
b. a contracted uterus.
c. a soft uterus.
d. decreased blood pressure.

16-22
C
Appl.
Impl.

A client and her husband plan on an early discharge from the hospital following the birth of their infant. Which would NOT be included in the immediate postpartal care of the client during the fourth stage of labor?

a. taking the blood pressure and pulse every 15 minutes
b. assessing for vaginal bleeding every 15 minutes
c. continuous massage of the fundus
d. palpating for bladder distention

16-23
C
Appl.
Impl.

A client has just delivered an infant vaginally. The heart rate is 100 BPM and the infant is crying vigorously with the limbs flexed. The infant's trunk is pink but the hands and feet are cyanotic. The infant cries when the soles of its feet are stimulated. The Apgar score for this infant would be:

a. 7.
b. 8.
c. 9.
d. 10.

16-24
B
Know.
Asses.

An infant's Apgar score is ascertained after birth at 1 minute and again at _____ minutes.

a. 5
b. 10
c. 11
d. 20

16-25
B
Appl.
Plan.

The first nursing action in caring for the newborn immediately after birth is:

a. maintenance of warmth.
b. maintenance of respirations.
c. identification of the newborn.
d. promotion of attachment.

16-26
D
Appl.
Asses.

In addition to the normal admission considerations for a laboring client, the nurse's PRIORITY assessment for an adolescent client should consider the client's:

a. cultural background.
b. plans to keep the infant.
c. support person.
d. developmental level.

16-27
B
Appl.
Impl.

The laboring client has delivered prior to the arrival of the physician. Which of the following nursing actions is MOST appropriate to decrease postpartal bleeding?

a. administering 10 units of Pitocin IM
b. putting the infant to breast
c. continuously massaging the fundus
d. inserting a perineal pad in the vagina

16-28
B
Comp.
Impl.

The Rileys have requested a Leboyer delivery. In supporting the Rileys, it is important for the nurse to:

a. clamp the cord immediately.
b. warm the bath water to 98 or 99 degrees F.
c. perform an immediate physical exam on the infant.
d. make sure the birthing area is well-lighted.

Chapter 17

Maternal Analgesia and Anesthesia

Instructions: For each of the following multiple-choice questions, select the ONE most appropriate answer.

Larry and Abbey Dean are admitted to the labor and delivery suite. Abbey has had a spontaneous rupture of membranes and is having mild contractions every 15 minutes for 30 seconds. The couple have completed a prepared childbirth course.

(THE FOLLOWING 10 ITEMS RELATE TO THE ABOVE PASSAGE.)

17-1
C
Appl.
Plan.

During the admission interview the couple tell the nurse they plan on having a medication-free birth. When discussing medication alternatives with Larry and Abbey the nurse's response should PRIMARILY focus on the fact that:

a. medication will only be offered if it is needed.
b. adequate pain relief will help the couple enjoy the birth experience.
c. maternal discomfort and anxiety may have more adverse effect on the fetus than a small amount of an analgesic agent.
d. medication will allow the laboring client to rest and not to be exhausted after the birth.

17-2
C
Comp.
Asses.

Abbey is not responding to her husband's coaching, can't relax, and is having difficulty keeping up with her breathing. Her last vaginal examination showed her to be 6 cm dilated, 100% effaced, and vertex presentation at 0 station. The nurse suggests some medication that might help her cope with her contractions. Abbey states, "I can manage without drugs." The nurse understands Abbey's refusal of medication may reflect:

a. noncompliance.
b. selfishness.
c. sense of inadequacy.
d. insecurity.

17-3
D
Comp.
Plan.

Which of the following is NOT criteria in the selection of analgesia for use during labor? The analgesia must:

a. provide maximum maternal analgesia.
b. be of minimum risk to the mother.
c. be of minimum risk to the fetus.
d. have no effect on uterine contractions.

17-4
A
Comp.
Plan.

After pointing out to the Deans that medication could help Abbey better use her breathing and participate more fully in the childbirth process, the couple agree to accept some medication. The drug classification MOST LIKELY to be used during the active phase of labor is:

a. narcotic analgesic.
b. opiate antagonist.
c. ataractic.
d. sedative.

17-5
C
Comp.
Analy.

Analgesia is not administered prior to the establishment of good labor PRIMARILY because it might:

a. cause fetal depression.
b. not be effective at the end of active labor.
c. prolong labor.
d. lead to maternal hypotension.

17-6
A
Know.
Plan.

The nurse obtains an order from the physician to give Abbey Demerol 25 mg. The preferred method of administering this drug is by which route?

a. intravenous
b. intramuscular
c. subcutaneous
d. oral

17-7
C
Know.
Asses.

The nurse applies the external fetal monitor to Abbey because s/he needs to assess the effects of the medication on:

a. Abbey's pain.
b. Abbey's physical status.
c. the labor contractions.
d. the fetus.

17-8
D
Comp.
Analy.

The nurse frequently assesses the laboring client's vital signs PRIMARILY because:

a. the administration of an analgesic agent is very likely to cause shock.
b. an increase in vital signs indicates that the mother is experiencing pain.
c. changes in vital signs tend to occur during a medicated labor.
d. any alteration in adequate functioning of the mother's cardiopulmonary system affects fetal well-being.

17-9
B
Appl.
Eval.

Abbey has received the Demerol. The nurse assesses the effectiveness of the medication PRIMARILY by assessing:

a. Abbey's vital signs.
b. Abbey's coping behavior with her uterine contractions.
c. the fetal heart rate variability.
d. the intensity of the uterine contractions.

17-10
C
Know.
Plan.

Abbey tells the nurse that she feels like pushing. A vaginal examination reveals a cervix that is completely dilated and the vertex is on the floor of the perineum. Abbey is about to deliver and it has been 1 hour since the administration of the Demerol. The drug of choice to reverse the effects of the narcotic analgesic would be:

a. Nisentil.
b. Valium.
c. Narcan.
d. Phenergan.

Donna Harbaugh is a gravida 2, para 1 client admitted in the active phase of labor. She tells the nurse, "I was so medicated for pain during my last labor and birth that I don't remember anything. I want to see and enjoy the birth this time."

(THE FOLLOWING 7 ITEMS RELATE TO THE ABOVE PASSAGE.)

17-11
A
Comp.
Plan.

The anesthesia which would best help Donna achieve her goal during the active phase of her labor would be:

a. paracervical.
b. pundendal.
c. spinal.
d. local infiltration.

17-12
B
Know.
Asses.

Donna is 5 cm dilated and completely effaced. Her physician decides an epidural anesthesia would best meet her needs. An epidural anesthetic is an example of what type of anesthesia?

a. intrathecal
b. regional
c. local
d. general

17-13
D
Appl.
Impl.

Donna's husband tells the nurse his sister had "medicine put in her back" when she had a baby and had a headache for a week afterwards. The nurse explains that the difference between the epidural and the spinal, in this regard, is that the spinal anesthetic:

a. can lead to hypertension which leads to a headache.
b. has a medication used with it that causes the headache.
c. lasts longer than the epidural so the side effects are greater.
d. penetrates the dura and allows the release of cerebrospinal fluid which leads to the headache.

17-14
D
Appl.
Impl.

Donna and her husband ask the nurse how this anesthesia is supposed to work. The nurse explains to the client:

a. "Medication will be injected into the spine to relieve the pain."
b. "Medication will be given to numb the area where the pain is coming from."
c. "Don't worry, you won't feel a thing."
d. "The medication is placed through a tube in your back, where it prevents the pain from the uterus from reaching your brain."

17-15
A
Appl.
Asses.

Following the injection of the anesthetic agent into the epidural catheter, the nurse checks for the effectiveness of the block by assessing for pain relief and:

a. increased temperature of the client's feet.
b. urinary retention.
c. decreased sensations of the upper extremities.
d. maternal headache.

17-16
A
Comp.
Asses.

Since Donna has had an epidural anesthetic, it is MOST important that the nurse assess for:

a. hypotension.
b. headache.
c. urinary retention.
d. hypoglycemia.

17-17
C
Appl.
Eval.

Since the local anesthetic agents used for epidural anesthesia only block certain fibers, the nurse should expect, during the second stage of labor, that Donna will most likely exhibit which type of behavior?

a. crying-out during contractions
b. falling asleep during contractions
c. pushing during contractions
d. ambulating during contractions

17-18
B
Know.
Plan.

The paracervical block only provides effective uterine pain relief during the first stage of labor because the anesthetic agent is injected into the:

a. pudendal nerves.
b. hypogastric plexus.
c. solar plexus.
d. uterine artery.

17-19
C
Appl.
Asses.

The adverse effects of using the paracervical block make it very important for the nurse to assess for:

a. maternal hypotension.
b. maternal allergic reactions.
c. fetal bradycardia.
d. fetal hemorrhage.

17-20
C
Comp.
Analy.

Which of the following is the DISADVANTAGE of using opiate-type drugs through an epidural route during the second stage of labor?

a. high incidence of nausea and vomiting
b. high incidence of pruritis
c. inadequate analgesia for delivery
d. respiratory depression

17-21
C
Know.
Plan.

The PRIMARY advantage of using inhalation anesthesia over intravenous anesthesia is that inhalation anesthesia is:

a. better tolerated by the client.
b. easier to administer.
c. easier to control the circulating concentration.
d. lower in the number of toxic effects.

17-22
A
Appl.
Impl.

The physician orders the administration of an inhalation anesthetic for cervical relaxation to facilitate forceps delivery of the fetus. Nursing actions would NOT include:

a. giving the client an antacid on the delivery table just prior to induction.
b. assessing the fetal heart rate during delivery.
c. maintaining the intravenous infusion.
d. maintaining uterine displacement until delivery.

17-23
B
Appl.
Impl.

The INITIAL responses of the nurse if the client aspires is to:

a. initiate suctioning of the nasooropharynx.
b. alter the delivery table to a Trendelenburg position.
c. turn the client to her side.
d. remove food particles from the oropharnyx.

17-24
C
Know.
Impl.

The PRIMARY nursing action to assist a woman experiencing preterm labor is to:

a. administer medication as ordered.
b. teach her proper breathing techniques.
c. provide emotional support.
d. monitor her vital signs.

17-25
A
Appl.
Asses.

After a cesarean delivery, under general anesthesia for a placenta previa, the nurse would continuously assess the client for clinical manifestations of which of the following complications of general anesthesia?

a. uterine atony
b. hypotension
c. vomiting
d. aspiration

17-26
D
Appl.
Impl.

The best nursing action to prevent heart failure in pregnancy-induced hypertension and cardiac clients while they receive regional anesthesia is to:

a. monitor the maternal blood pressure.
b. position the client appropriately.
c. decrease the amount of intravenous fluid infusing.
d. monitor the central venous pressure.

17-27
A
Appl.
Impl.

A nursing action which would ease the induction of general anesthesia in obstetrical clients requiring emergency surgical intervention would be to:

a. provide the client with a simple, concise explanation.
b. prepare the client as quickly as possible for surgery.
c. administer sedation as quickly as possible.
d. allow the couple time alone together.

17-28 Lois Hudson is in labor with her third child and has requested an epidural
B   anesthetic. Lois asks the nurse, "When can I have the epidural?" The nurse
Comp. explains that it can be given:
Impl.

    a. immediately before Lois is taken to the delivery.
    b. when active labor has been established.
    c. whenever Lois wants it.
    d. when Lois enters the transition phase.

17-29 To evaluate Lois for the most likely side effects of the epidural, the nurse should
A   monitor her:
Know.
Impl. a. blood pressure.
    b. respiratory rate.
    c. tendon reflexes.
    d. urine output.

Chapter 18

Intrapartal Family at Risk

Instructions: For each of the following multiple-choice questions, select the ONE most appropriate answer.

Myrna Fields, a 33-year-old multigravida, was admitted to the hospital in the active ～～ of labor. During the admission assessment, Myrna tells the nurse she had ～～me bright red bleeding since her contractions began.

NG 5 ITEMS RELATE TO THE ABOVE PASSAGE.)

.r/his assessment of Myrna, the nurse should omit:

na's vital signs.
.g for fetal heart tones.
.g cervical effacement and dilation.
frequency, intensity, and duration of contractions.

... reasons for vaginal bleeding during the intrapartal period are abruptio ～～a and placenta previa. Which of the following manifestations would be MOST indicative of abruptio placenta?

a. maternal hypotension
b. fetal distress
c. pain
d. decreased hemoglobin

18-3
D
Comp.
Asses.

The nurse monitors maternal vital signs at frequent intervals. Her/his PRIMARY reason for this action is to assess for the presence of:

a. anxiety.
b. hypertension.
c. discomfort.
d. hemorrhage.

18-4
C
Comp.
Plan.

The best method of assessing fetal response at this time is by using the:

a. fetoscope.
b. doppler stethoscope.
c. external monitor.
d. internal monitor.

18-5
C
Appl.
Impl.

The physician diagnoses a total placenta previa. S/he explains the situation to Myrna and leaves to arrange for a cesarean birth. Myrna's eyes are filled with tears. The MOST appropriate nursing action at this time is to:

a. ask the physician to come back and talk with Myrna again.
b. ask Myrna if she has a family member you can contact.
c. take Myrna's hand.
d. start to gather the equipment to prepare for the cesarean birth.

Deborah Frasier is a 36-year-old multigravida who has just delivered twin girls by section after a failed oxytocin augmentation. Deborah has an antepartal history of pregnancy-induced hypertension. The physician discovered a marginal sinus rupture of the placenta. Deborah remains in the recovery room of the labor and delivery suite 3 hours after birth because she cannot adequately control her legs following the termination of the epidural anesthesia.

(THE FOLLOWING 5 ITEMS RELATE TO THE ABOVE PASSAGE.)

18-6
C
Comp.
Asses

While repositioning Deborah, the nurse notices that the site of the epidural injection is oozing. The nurse suspects disseminating intravascular coagulation (DIC). What other clinical manifestation of DIC would the nurse be MOST likely to find?

a. epistaxis
b. petechiae on the legs
c. increased vaginal bleeding
d. bleeding gums

18-7
B
Comp.
Analy.

The nurse notifies the physician who orders the appropriate blood test. Which of the following results would be indicative of DIC?

a. increased platelet count
b. prolonged partial thromboplastin time
c. increased fibrinogen level
d. decreased hemoglobin

18-8
D
Comp.
Asses.

What other risk factor can be identified in Deborah's history that might predispose her to the development of DIC?

a. twin pregnancy
b. cesarean birth
c. multiparity
d. pregnancy-induced hypertension

18-9
C
Know.
Impl.

The nurse would MOST likely receive orders to administer which of the following agents to treat the absence of clotting factors which occurs in DIC?

a. packed cells
b. plasmanate
c. cryoprecipitate
d. heparin

18-10
B
Appl.
Plan.

In planning care for Deborah, which of the following would NOT be included?

a. frequent assessment of vital signs
b. administration of intramuscular injections of analgesics
c. administration of blood products
d. observation of hourly urinary output

Edith Bryant is a primigravida admitted to the hospital in early labor. She is 3 cm dilated, head at -2 station with intact membranes. The fetal heart rate is 154 by auscultation with the fetoscope. About an hour after admission Edith has a spontaneous rupture of membranes.

(THE FOLLOWING 4 ITEMS RELATE TO THE ABOVE PASSAGE.)

18-11
C
Appl.
Impl.

After the initial action of auscultating the fetal heart rate, the nurse should:

a. assess present cervical dilation.
b. palpate for frequency, intensity, and duration of contractions.
c. auscultate the FHR after the next few contractions.
d. document the client's response to the amniotomy.

18-12
D
Appl.
Impl.

The nurse sees a change in the FHR to 100 BPM with moderate variable decelerations. The INITIAL nursing response should be to:

a. administer oxygen per nasal cannula.
b. alter the client's position in bed.
c. notify the physician.
d. perform a vaginal examination.

18-13
D
Comp.
Analy.

During a vaginal exam, the nurse palpates a loop of prolapsed umbilical cord beside the fetal head. The nurse has Edith's husband assist Edith into a knee-chest position while s/he keeps her/his hand in the vagina. The rationale for this action is to:

a. help the fetal head descend faster.
b. prevent head compression during contractions.
c. facilitate rapid dilation of the cervix.
d. relieve compression of the cord through gravity and manipulation.

18-14
C
Appl.
Impl.

An emergency cesarean section is performed under general anesthesia but the infant is stillborn. Which of the following nursing actions would NOT facilitate the grief process for the Bryants?

a. Encourage the parents to express their feelings to each other.
b. Allow the parents to see their baby if they wish.
c. Leave the couple alone so that they can express their grief in private.
d. Furnish the parents with a community support referral.

Delia Jenkins arrives at the labor and delivery suite with her husband, Jay. This is her first baby, and she states her contractions are every 4 to 5 minutes and last about 45 seconds. She and her husband have completed a prepared childbirth class. She says that her contractions are very painful and that they tense her body. She grimaces with each contraction.

(THE FOLLOWING 2 ITEMS RELATE TO THE ABOVE PASSAGE.)

18-15
C
Comp.
Analy.
During the admission procedure, the nurse continues to observe Delia for manifestations of anxiety. Which of the following statements MOST completely describes the relationship between anxiety and labor?

a. Increased utilization of glucose stores, caused by stress and anxiety, decrease the availability of glucose to the contracting uterus.
b. Peripheral vasoconstriction, caused by norepinephrine, decreases the blood supply to the contracting uterus.
c. Anxiety, fear, and labor pain result in catecholamine release which can ultimately result in myometrial dysfunction and ineffectual labor.
d. Epinephrine inhibits myometrial activity and therefore uterine contractility.

18-16
B
Comp.
Diag.
Delia continues to exhibit a high degree of muscle tension even without contractions. She is not able to follow her husband's instructions to relax and breathe. The nurse makes the diagnosis of:

a. fear.
b. ineffective individual coping.
c. anxiety.
d. knowledge deficit.

Delia Jenkins' cervical status remains unchanged 3 hours after admission. The fetal heart rate is now 160 BPM. The contractions are every 5 to 7 minutes and last 30 seconds. The physician diagnoses dysfunctional hypotonic labor pattern. After satisfactory pelvimetry results, the physician performs an amniotomy and orders an oxytocin augmentation.

(THE FOLLOWING 3 ITEMS RELATE TO THE ABOVE PASSAGE.)

18-17
B
Know.
Asses.
Which of the following statements is NOT associated with a hypotonic labor pattern?

a. Contractions decrease in quality and frequency.
b. Sedation is effective in relieving the condition.
c. The client responds favorably to oxytocin.
d. The condition is most often seen in the active phase of labor.

18-18
C
Appl.
Impl.
The internal monitor for both fetal heart rate and uterine contractions is applied. The nurse assesses late decelerations. The nurse's INITIAL action is to:

a. change maternal position.
b. administer oxygen by mouth.
c. discontinue oxytocin infusion.
d. notify the physician.

18-19
A
Know.
Plan.
The complication, common to both the mother and fetus, resulting from a prolonged labor is:

a. infection.
b. hemorrhage.
c. cerebral trauma.
d. hypovolemia.

18-20
D
Know.
Asses.

Precipitous labor is one that:

a. occurs without the mother's awareness.
b. occurs before the expected date of birth.
c. is of 2 hours' duration or less.
d. is of 3 hours' duration or less.

18-21
B
Appl.
Impl.

During a precipitous delivery it is MOST important for the nurse NOT to:

a. take time to cleanse her/his hands to prevent infection.
b. position the mother to prevent delivery.
c. remove amniotic fluid from the infant's oronasalpharynx.
d. prepare a sterile field for the delivery.

18-22
B
Appl.
Impl.

While giving care to a client experiencing premature rupture of membranes, the nurse would OMIT which of the following nursing actions?

a. monitoring the occurrence of uterine contractions
b. performing frequent, sterile, vaginal examinations to assess cervical status
c. monitoring fetal heart rate and maternal vital signs
d. observing white blood cell count

18-23
D
Know.
Analy.

The critical factor which increases mortality for neonates born before 37 weeks' gestation is the neonate's:

a. insufficient fat storage.
b. inability to maintain body heat.
c. immature digestive system.
d. underdeveloped respiratory system.

18-24
A
Appl.
Asses.

For a client with a diagnosis of premature labor who is receiving a beta-adrenergic agent to inhibit labor, it is critical that the nurse assess which body system?

a. cardiovascular
b. endocrine
c. circulatory
d. nervous

18-25
D
Appl.
Impl.

The nurse may help a client rotate a fetus that is in a persistent left occiput posterior position by:

a. having the woman assume a dorsal recumbent position.
b. applying counterpressure in the sacral area.
c. helping the client ambulate during early labor.
d. having the client assume a knee-chest position.

18-26
C
Appl.
Impl.

The client vaginally delivers an infant weighing 4750 g. During her/his initial assessment the nurse looks for:

a. Bell's palsy.
b. bradycardia.
c. Erb's palsy.
d. petechiae.

Chapter 19

Obstetric Procedures: The Role of the Nurse

Instructions: For each of the following multiple-choice questions, select the ONE most appropriate answer.

19-1
B
Know.
Analy.

There has been an increase in cesarean births in recent years for all of the following reasons EXCEPT:

a. there are better diagnostic techniques available.
b. the woman can spend more time with her child before returning to work.
c. obstetric philosophy is turning toward more rapid interventions in the labor process.
d. the procedure itself is safer than in the past.

19-2
D
Comp.
Diag.

Cesarean birth would be an appropriate choice for:

a. Mrs. Jones, who fears natural childbirth.
b. Mrs. Smith, who has a history of hypertension.
c. Mrs. Locke, who has a low pain threshold.
d. Mrs. Rich, who has a cephalopelvic disproportion.

19-3
D
Know.
Analy.

The alteration of fetal position by abdominal or intrauterine manipulation to accomplish a more favorable fetal position is termed:

a. amniotomy.
b. Leopold's maneuver.
c. ballottement.
d. version.

19-4
A
Comp.
Analy.

The prerequisites for cephalic version include all of the following EXCEPT:

a. the presenting part must be engaged.
b. the uterine wall must not be irritable.
c. the membranes must be intact.
d. there must be a sufficient quantity of amniotic fluid.

Cheryl Tigert has been admitted for a cephalic version. She has just returned from ultrasound and a fetal heart monitor has been attached.

(THE FOLLOWING 2 ITEMS RELATE TO THE ABOVE PASSAGE.)

19-5
D
Comp.
Impl.

Cheryl's obstetrician has ordered intravenous Ritodrine for the purpose of:

a. providing maternal analgesia.
b. inducing labor.
c. preventing hemorrhage.
d. achieving uterine relaxation.

19-6
A
Appl.
Impl.

During the version process, Cheryl begins to scream and toss about. The most appropriate intervention is to:

a. discontinue the version procedure.
b. begin coaching her in breathing techniques.
c. obtain an order for a non-narcotic analgesic.
d. put on some music for distraction.

19-7
C
Know.
Asses.

The MOST common operative obstetric procedure is:

a. cesarean birth.
b. episiotomy.
c. amniotomy.
d. internal version.

19-8
B
Comp.
Analy.

Internal (podalic) version is attempted in:

a. adolescents with a breech presentation.
b. multiple gestations for birth of the second twin.
c. obstetric intensive care units only.
d. response to fetal distress.

Nancy Long, 27 years old, is admitted to the labor and delivery unit in the early a.m. Her obstetrician has suggested an amniotomy as a method of labor induction.

(THE FOLLOWING 3 ITEMS RELATE TO THE ABOVE PASSAGE.)

19-9
C
Comp.
Analy.

Advantages of amniotomy as a method of labor induction include all of the following EXCEPT:

a. contractions are similar to spontaneous labor.
b. there is little risk of a ruptured uterus.
c. the danger of a prolapsed cord is decreased.
d. fetal monitoring is facilitated.

19-10
C
Comp.
Analy.

Disadvantages of amniotomy include all of the following EXCEPT:

a. birth must occur even if subsequent findings suggest delay.
b. the risk of infection is increased.
c. there is risk of hypertonia and uterine rupture.
d. compression and molding of the fetal head increases.

19-11
A
Comp.
Asses.

Before amniotomy is performed, the fetus is assessed for all of the following EXCEPT:

a. estimated birth weight.
b. presentation.
c. station.
d. position.

19-12
A
Comp.
Analy.

Unless the head is well-engaged in the pelvis, dangers associated with an amniotomy include all of the following EXCEPT:

a. sudden cessation of labor.
b. prolapsed cord.
c. abruptio placenta.
d. amniotic fluid embolus.

Patricia Nicholson, 22 years old, requires induced labor.

(THE FOLLOWING 4 ITEMS RELATE TO THE ABOVE PASSAGE.)

19-13
D
Comp.
Asses.

Prior to an elective induction of labor it is essential to determine:

a. the mother's Rh factor.
b. fetal heart rate.
c. station and presentation.
d. gestational dating.

19-14
B
Comp.
Impl.

Indications for induction of labor include all of the following EXCEPT:

a. chronic hypertension.
b. schizophrenia or manic-depressive psychoses.
c. renal disease.
d. diabetes mellitus.

19-15
A
Comp.
Impl.

The MOST important criterion for successful induction of labor is:

a. cervical readiness.
b. stable maternal vital signs.
c. adequate fetal position and station.
d. willingness of family for induction.

19-16
D
Know.
Plan.

A nurse is preparing a teaching pamphlet on oxytocin induction. Which of the following statements might be included regarding risks?

a. There is no increased risk of uterine rupture.
b. Cervical and/or perineal laceration frequently occur.
c. Irritability of the bladder is common.
d. Oxytocin induction may cause hyperstimulation of the uterus.

19-17
C
Comp.
Eval.

You are assisting in an oxytocin induction and are infusing 28 mU/min. of oxytocin. You would be especially alert for signs of:

a. hypoglycemic shock.
b. uterine rupture.
c. water intoxication.
d. maternal hemorrhage.

19-18
B
Appl.
Impl.

If administered within 2 to 4 hours before birth, analgesia:

a. may serve the same purpose as preoperative sedation.
b. may result in neonatal respiratory distress.
c. may enhance the delivery process.
d. may prevent the need for an episiotomy.

19-19
A
Comp.
Diag.

Water intoxication may be manifested by all of the following EXCEPT:

a. hypertension.
b. cardiac arrhythmias.
c. nausea and/or vomiting.
d. mental confusion.

19-20
D
Comp.
Impl.

It is important that the nurse discontinue an oxytocin infusion in all of the following situations EXCEPT when:

a. the woman's contractions are more frequent than 2 minutes.
b. contraction duration exceeds 90 seconds.
c. the uterus does not relax between contractions.
d. the woman complains of increasing discomfort.

19-21
C
Comp.
Impl.

An episiotomy may be performed for all of the following reasons EXCEPT:

a. to minimize stretching of perineal tissue.
b. to decrease incidence of perineal lacerations.
c. to minimize duration of labor.
d. to decrease trauma to fetal head during birth.

19-22
B
Comp.
Impl.

Indications for the use of forceps during delivery include all of the following EXCEPT:

a. threat to the life of mother or fetus.
b. desire for a more rapid delivery.
c. prolapsed cord.
d. maternal exhaustion.

19-23
B
Comp.
Impl.

Which of the following meets prerequisites for low forceps birth?

a. A primipara who is 8 centimeters dilated and completely effaced.
b. A multipara who is completely dilated and effaced and the fetal vertex is on the perineum.
c. A fetus is in breech presentation and at -1 station.
d. Amniotic membranes are bulging.

19-24
A
Know.
Impl.

The most common indication for the use of a vacuum extractor is:

a. prolongation of the second stage of labor.
b. prevention of maternal hemorrhage.
c. prevention of fetal abnormalities.
d. prolongation of the first stage of labor.

19-25
C
Know.
Asses.

The type of cesarean incision made across the lowest and narrowest part of the abdomen is called a _____ incision.

a. vertical
b. suprapubic
c. transverse
d. horizontal

19-26
A
Know.
Asses.

The type of incision that is preferred for a cesarean birth is the:

a. transverse incision.
b. vertical incision.
c. horizontal incision.
d. suprapubic incision.

19-27
A
Know.
Asses.

The current incidence of cesarean births is believed to be:

a. 1 in 5.
b. 1 in 10.
c. 1 in 15.
d. 1 in 30.

Kathy Slaubaugh, gravida 2, para 1, is 2 weeks past her estimated due date, and she has been admitted for possible induction of labor. Her husband, Charles, is with her. She has had no problems with her pregnancy.

(THE FOLLOWING 5 ITEMS RELATE TO THE ABOVE PASSAGE.)

19-28
C
Comp.
Analy.

After analyzing the initial assessment data, the nurse knows that a contraindication for induction is:

a. a previous birth
b. young maternal age (under 20)
c. central placenta previa.
d. vertex presentation.

19-29
A
Appl.
Impl.

Kathy and Charles state that they were told about inductions in their childbirth classes, but that they wonder whether this labor will be shorter than the previous time. The nurse's best initial response should be:

a. "Length of labor depends on many factors."
b. "Induced labors are usually longer."
c. "Induced labors are always shorter."
d. "Don't worry. The doctor will take care of everything."

19-30
C
Appl.
Plan.

In planning nursing care for Kathy, the nurse makes provision for:

a. frequent ambulation.
b. limited visiting privileges for Charles.
c. assessing maternal vital signs every 15 minutes.
d. evaluating fetal blood gases every 2 hours.

19-31
D
Comp.
Impl.

One of the nurse's actions during Kathy's induction is closely recording her intake and output. This is to help monitor for the oxytocin side effect of:

a. uterine hyperstimulation.
b. hypertension.
c. hypotension.
d. water intoxication.

19-32
C
Comp.
Impl.

When palpating Kathy's fundus after birth, the nurse discovers that it is not firm. The nurse's first action would be to:

a. notify the physician.
b. increase the flow rate of the IV.
c. massage the fundus.
d. elevate Kathy's hips.

Instructions: For each of the following multiple-choice questions, select the ONE most appropriate answer.

20-1
D
Know.
Asses.

Which two neonatal body systems must undergo the MOST RAPID changes to support extrauterine life?

a. gastrointestinal and hepatic
b. urinary and hematologic
c. neurologic and temperature control
d. respiratory and cardiovascular

Kathy is a term newborn who experienced no respiratory distress at birth.

(THE FOLLOWING 11 ITEMS RELATE TO THE ABOVE PASSAGE.)

20-2
C
Appl.
Asses.

Kathy's lecithin to sphingomyelin ratio (L/S ratio) at at the time of birth was MOST probably:

a. 1:1.
b. less than 1:1.
c. 2:1 or greater.
d. too low to be measurable.

20-3
A
Comp.
Asses.

The fluid in Kathy's lungs prior to birth originated:

a. from secretions produced by the fetal lungs.
b. in secretions aspirated from the birth canal.
c. from swallowed amniotic fluid.
d. in capillary fluid which osmosed into the fetal lungs.

20-4
B
Appl.
Diag.

Which of the following situations related to Kathy's birth would have affected the PRIMARY mechanism of MECHANICAL fluid removal from her lungs?

a. administration of oxygen via face mask
b. delivery via cesarean birth
c. failure to cry at birth
d. low serum protein level

20-5
D
Comp.
Impl.

At birth a DeLee device was used with Kathy. The purpose of this was to:

a. expand the alveoli.
b. increase available oxygen.
c. decompress the stomach.
d. remove fluid from the oropharynx.

20-6
A
Know.
Diag.

The onset of Kathy's breathing was chemically stimulated by which normal, transitory, blood gas alteration?

a. acidosis
b. alkalosis
c. increased pO_2
d. decreased pCO_2

20-7
B
Appl.
Asses.

If Kathy had been born with a surfactant deficit, the nurse would most likely observe:

a. jaundice.
b. sternal retractions.
c. abdominal distention.
d. frothy, blood-tinged sputum.

20-8
C
Know.
Diag.

Air entering Kathy's lungs immediately after birth effects cardiopulmonary physiology by:

a. decreasing pulmonary blood flow and increasing alveolar pCO_2 levels.
b. increasing alveolar pO_2 and pulmonary vascular resistance.
c. increasing alveolar pO_2 and decreasing pulmonary vascular resistance.
d. increasing pulmonary blood flow and pCO_2 levels.

20-9
C
Appl.
Asses.

Because of the high levels of fetal hemoglobin (Hgb F) present in the neonatal period, it is important for the nurse to know that Kathy:

a. exhibits the usual clinical signs of hypoxia readily.
b. has greater oxygen available to the tissues than an adult.
c. will not exhibit cyanosis as readily when O_2 blood levels drop.
d. will exhibit cyanosis at relatively high blood oxygen levels.

20-10
A
Appl.
Impl.

At 12 hours of age, Kathy's respiratory rate is 44 per minute. Her respirations are shallow with periods of apnea lasting up to 5 seconds. Based upon this assessment data the nurse should:

a. continue routine monitoring.
b. activate respiratory arrest procedures.
c. request an order for supplemental oxygen.
d. call the clinician immediately and report her/his assessment.

20-11
D
Appl.
Impl.

Placement of a nasogastric tube in a neonate such as Kathy can result in severe respiratory distress if:

a. bolus rather than continuous feeding are initiated via the tube.
b. the tube is taped to the infant's forehead.
c. the tube enters the duodenum.
d. the nonintubated nare becomes occluded.

20-12
D
Know.
Diag.

Closure of Kathy's foramen ovale occurs when:

a. the umbilical cord is severed.
b. blood flows from the pulmonary artery to the aorta.
c. increased pO_2 causes constriction to occur.
d. left atrial pressure exceeds right atrial pressure.

Zoe Dumas is a 2-day-old, full-term neonate. To this point, Zoe's neonatal course has been uneventful.

(THE FOLLOWING 10 ITEMS RELATE TO THE ABOVE PASSAGE.)

20-13
B
Know.
Asses.

In assessing Zoe's heart rate the nurse should:

a. palpate the carotid artery for 1 minute.
b. auscultate the apical rate for 1 minute.
c. palpate the radial pulse for 30 seconds and multiply by 2.
d. auscultate the apical rate for 15 seconds and multiply by 4.

20-14
A
Comp.
Eval.

If Zoe's vital signs are taken during a crying episode, the nurse would expect to find:

a. an elevated heart rate and blood pressure.
b. an elevated heart rate and decreased blood pressure.
c. a decreased heart rate and blood pressure.
d. a decreased heart rate and increased blood pressure.

20-15
B
Appl.
Asses.

Zoe's mother is alarmed when the doctor states s/he heard a heart murmur when auscultating Zoe's chest. Later that morning Zoe's mother questions the nurse for clarification. Which statement by the nurse is most consistent with current knowledge of heart murmurs in the neonatal period?

a. "All babies have heart murmurs. Don't worry about Zoe."
b. "Most heart murmurs in young babies are not serious and disappear in a short time."
c. "Zoe most likely has a hole in her heart."
d. "Zoe will be transferred to the neonatal ICU so we can monitor her heart murmur."

20-16
B
Appl.
Eval.

Zoe's blood tests in the first few days of life should reveal hemoglobin and hematocrit values:

a. lower than comparable adult values.
b. consistent with active fetal erythropoiesis.
c. demonstrating shift of fluid to the intravascular compartment.
d. consistent with high O_2 fetal oxygen saturation.

20-17
C
Comp.
Plan.

In relationship to adults, Zoe's ability to maintain a thermoneutral environment requires:

a. higher environmental oxygen levels.
b. greater relative muscle mass.
c. higher environmental temperatures.
d. environmental temperatures and oxygen levels greater than the adult's.

20-18
A
Know.
Appl.

Temperature instability in neonates such as Zoe is primarily the result of:

a. excessive heat loss.
b. impaired thermogenesis.
c. immature central control (hypothalamus).
d. lack of glycogen stores.

20-19
A
Comp.
Diag.

Which of the following physical characteristics serves to decrease Zoe's loss of heat?

a. flexed posture
b. blood vessel dilatation
c. limited subcutaneous fat
d. larger body surface relative to an adult's

20-20
A
Comp.
Impl.

Zoe's body temperature drops when she is placed on the cool, plastic surface of an infant seat. This is an example of heat loss via:

a. conduction.
b. convection.
c. evaporation.
d. radiation.

20-21
C
Appl.
Impl.

If Zoe's blood glucose level is 40mg/dL on the third day after birth, the nurse should:

a. recognize this as a normal value.
b. observe for clinical signs of hyperglycemia.
c. institute the nursery policy for the hypoglycemic infant.
d. substitute sterile water feedings instead of formula.

20-22
B
Appl.
Impl.

On the third day after birth, Zoe's skin turns a yellow color. Zoe's mother asks the nurse if Zoe has "that contagious liver disease." The most appropriate nursing response in terms of meeting the mother's emotional and knowledge needs is:

a. "Don't be silly, you know that Zoe hasn't received a blood transfusion."
b. "I can tell that you are worried about Zoe. Let me talk to you about this temporary change in Zoe's condition."
c. "Just let me worry about Zoe's skin color -- you concentrate on learning how to bathe and feed her."
d. "We will be isolating Zoe for a few days until her skin is no longer yellow. She has a condition known as physiologic jaundice."

20-23
D
Comp.
Impl.

Vitamin K (Aquamephyton) is administered to newborns to:

a. stimulate growth of intestinal flora.
b. promote absorption of fat-soluble nutrients.
c. speed conjugation of bilirubin.
d. prevent potential bleeding problems.

20-24   When compared to an adult's, the stools of a neonate contain more:
C
Comp.   a. glucose.
Diag.   b. protein.
         c. fat.
         d. maltose.

20-25   A newborn's mother is alarmed to find small amounts of blood on her infant's
D   diaper. When the nurse checks the female infant's urine it is straw-colored and
Appl.   has no offensive odor. Which explanation to the newborn's mother is most
Impl.   appropriate?

         a. "It appears your baby has a kidney infection."
         b. "Breast-fed babies often experience this type of bleeding problem due to lack
            of vitamin K in the breast milk."
         c. "The baby probably passed a small urate kidney stone."
         d. "Some infants experience menstruation-like bleeding when hormones from
            the mother are not available."

20-26   A neonate's father expresses concern that his baby does not have good control of
A   his hands and arms. It is important for the father to realize certain neurological
Comp.   patterns in the newborn such as:
Asses.
         a. function progresses in a head-to-toe, proximal-distal fashion.
         b. purposeless, uncoordinated movements of the arms are abnormal.
         c. mild hypotonia is expected in the upper extremities.
         d. asymmetric muscle tone is not unusual.

Flo Adams is admitted to the antepartal unit for observation. She is 30 weeks into
her pregnancy, and care is directed at prolonging the gestation period.

(THE FOLLOWING 3 ITEMS RELATE TO THE ABOVE PASSAGE.)

20-27   The nurse knows that if Flo's baby were delivered at 30 weeks' gestation, the
B   greatest threat to it's well-being would be:
Comp.
Asses.   a. inadequate thermal stimuli.
         b. lack of adequate surfactant.
         c. pronounced thrombocytopenia.
         d. reduced capillary permeability.

20-28   Substantial demands will be placed on Flo's baby, including cardiovascular
D   changes. Pulmonary vascular circulation in the neonate increases to 100% within:
Know.
Asses.   a. 1 hour after birth.
         b. 4 hours after birth.
         c. 12 hours after birth.
         d. 24 hours after birth.

114

20-29
C
Know.
Asses.

Baby Adams is delivered at 38 weeks' gestation. In the birthing room the nurse counts his respiratory rate and finds it it to be within the normal range of:

a. 18 to 22 breaths per minute.
b. 20 to 40 breaths per minute.
c. 30 to 50 breaths per minute.
d. 50 to 70 breaths per minute.

Chapter 21

Nursing Assessment of the Newborn

Instructions: For each of the following multiple-choice questions, select the ONE most appropriate answer.

21-1
C
Appl.
Plan.

Of the following information, which would be MOST important to note as part of the initial newborn assessment?

a. maternal age - 22 years
b. maternal smoking behavior - nonsmoker
c. maternal analgesia - Demerol 25 mg. IV, 15 min. prior to birth
d. maternal dietary intake - last meal 4 hours prior to initiation of active labor

Jason Monroe is a newborn male born in a hospital setting.

(THE FOLLOWING 8 ITEMS RELATE TO THE ABOVE PASSAGE.)

21-2
C
Comp.
Asses.

Jason's most complete newborn physical examination will occur:

a. in the delivery room at birth.
b. in the nursery during the first 4 hours.
c. in the nursery prior to discharge from the hospital.
d. in the physician's office at the 4 week follow-up appointment.

21-3
A
Know.
Impl.

Involvement of Jason's parents in the newborn nursing assessment process should begin:

a. in the birthing room.
b. when Jason is alone with his parents on the post-partum unit.
c. when the nurse reports her/his gestational age assessment to the parents.
d. after the three-phase, medical-nursing assessment process is completed.

21-4
A
Comp.
Impl.

The PRIMARY purpose for including Jason's parents in the assessment process is to:

a. promote parental-newborn attachment.
b. foster parental independence in providing Jason's care.
c. involve Jason's parents in decision making regarding his medical care.
d. support positive attitudes towards Jason's on-going health care.

21-5
D
Comp.
Asses.

Gestational age assessment is completed on Jason during the first four hours after birth because:

a. the physical criteria which are evaluated change rapidly after birth.
b. effects of labor and birth are least notable during this time frame.
c. separation from the parents is easily accomplished at this time.
d. age-related neonatal problems must be assessed and managed promptly.

21-6
B
Appl.
Asses.

Which of the following physical assessment data is LEAST reliable during the first four hours of Jason's life?

a. visible, abundant lanugo
b. positive Babinski reflex
c. descended testes with good rugae present
d. palpable, thick ear cartilage

21-7
A
Comp.
Asses.

The nurse documents Jason's physical characteristics. Which documentation is normally recorded as part of the gestation age assessment?

a. plantar creases present on anterior 2/3 of sole
b. umbilical cord moist to touch
c. anterior and posterior fontanels patent
d. milia present on bridge of nose

21-8
B
Comp.
Diag.

In estimating Jason's gestational age, it is important to remember that assessment criteria:

a. must correlate with the composite score to be useful.
b. may be affected by specific maternal health conditions.
c. are sometimes more accurate in assessing gestational age than the total score.
d. are more useful in assessing postmaturity than prematurity.

21-9
D
Know.
Diag.

The nurse notes that Jason's breast tissue consists of a flat areola with no bud. This finding is consistent with:

a. male gender.
b. a birth defect.
c. decreased maternal hormones.
d. preterm gestational age.

21-10
A
Appl.
Diag.

In the preterm newborn a finding of greater neuromuscular tone in the lower extremities than in the upper extremities MOST commonly indicates:

a. a normal gestational development pattern.
b. evidence of cephalocaudal fetal development.
c. cerebral palsy affecting the motor cortex.
d. abnormal intrauterine positioning prior to birth.

21-11
C
Know.
Asses.

The square window sign is elicited by:

a. flexing the foot toward the shin.
b. flexing the thigh on the abdomen.
c. flexing the hand toward the ventral forearm.
d. drawing the arm across the chest toward the opposite shoulder.

21-12 The nurse would expect to find a postmature newborn capable of:
D
Comp. a. ankle dorsiflexion to a 45 degree angle.
Asses. b. a 90 degree square window sign.
       c. moving the elbow past the midline of the body when the arm is pulled across
          the chest.
       d. keeping the head in front of the body when pulled to a sitting position.

Mike Wilson is a Caucasian infant born at term. He is the first-born child and his
parents are very anxious. Mike's birth weight was 3405 grams (7 lbs, 8 oz).

(THE FOLLOWING 5 ITEMS RELATE TO THE ABOVE PASSAGE.)

21-13 Mike's weight has dropped to 3361 grams by day three of his life. His parents are
C   very upset and question Mike's care in the nursery. Which of the following
Appl. statements by the nurse would be most therapeutic?
Impl.
       a. "All newborn babies lose weight."
       b. "I share your concern; Mike's weight loss is excessive."
       c. "I can see that you are very worried about Mike. This weight loss is an expected
          one and he will begin to gain weight now."
       d. "Mike eats well in the nursery; maybe you aren't feeding him properly. Show
          me how you feed him."

21-14 Mike's parents question how rapidly he should grow. Which response demonstrates
B   knowledge of the expected weight gain for the normal neonate?
Appl.
Impl. a. "Mike should triple his birth weight by the age of 6 months."
       b. "Mike should gain about 10 pounds during the next 6 months."
       c. "Most infants gain a pound a month for the first 6 months."
       d. none of these

21-15 Mike's mother asks why he always keeps his hands clenched and his knees and
A   elbows bent. The nurse's response should be based on the knowledge that:
Comp.
Impl. a. flexion is the normal position for the newborn.
       b. parental anxiety causes Mike's tension and flexed posture.
       c. placing Mike in a supine position will decrease his flexed posture.
       d. Mike's muscle tone will decrease when he is stimulated appropriately.

21-16 Of the following physical examination findings, which one should be immediately
D   reported to the clinician should Mike exhibit it?
Comp.
Asses. a. overriding cranial bones
       b. patent posterior fontanel
       c. spongy, edematous area of the scalp
       d. head circumference 4 cm. less than chest circumference

21-17 The nurse uses her/his fingertip to press Mike's gum line. S/he is assessing for:
B
Appl. a. presence of tooth buds.
Asses. b. evidence of increased bilirubin.
       c. adequacy of tissue perfusion.
       d. Mike's response to painful stimuli.

21-18   To obtain an infant's abdominal circumference, you would measure:
B
Know.   a. around the largest area.
Asses. b. at the level of the umbilicus.
        c. 5 cm. below the xiphoid process.
        d. with the infant in a sitting position.

Marie Valdez is a 2-day-old newborn. Marie's mother was exposed to rubella during her last pregnancy and is very anxious about the health of her newborn infant. Marie's mother is also concerned that Marie sheds no tears when she cries.

(THE FOLLOWING 4 ITEMS RELATE TO THE ABOVE PASSAGE.)

21-19   Marie's mother questions the nurse about Marie's absence of tears. The nurse's
D   response should be based on the knowledge that:
Comp.
Diag.   a. newborn lacrimal ducts must be punctured to initiate tear flow.
        b. silver nitrate instillation at birth reduces tear formation for several days.
        c. exposure to rubella in utero results in lacrimal duct stenosis.
        d. lacrimal ducts are usually nonfunctional until two months of age.

21-20   The nurse carefully assesses Marie's pupils for opacities. Her/his rationale for doing
C   this is because:
Appl.
Diag.   a. chemical conjunctivitis affects lens structure.
        b. eye hemorrhages manifest themselves as lens cloudiness.
        c. maternal history indicates rubella exposure.
        d. lack of tear production signifies eye abnormality.

21-21   Marie's hard and soft palate are palpated by the nurse's clean index finger. This
B   assessment is done to detect:
Comp.
Asses. a. sucking capability.
        b. openings in the palate.
        c. candida albicans infection.
        d. adequacy of saliva production.

21-22   Of the following assessments, which indicates an abnormal finding for Marie?
C
Comp.   a. cylindrical, protruding abdomen
Asses. b. blinking in response to bright light
        c. ability to sleep in presence of loud noises
        d. parallel relationship of top of ear to outer ear canthus

21-23   A nurse detects that a 5-day-old infant's femoral pulses are weaker than her brachial
D   pulses. The nurse's next intervention should be to assess:
Appl.
Impl.   a. time of last voiding.
        b. presence of bowel sounds.
        c. position of apical impulse.
        d. upper and lower extremity blood pressures.

21-24
C
Know.
Asses.

Which clinical manifestation is considered a normal finding related to the umbilical cord of a 4-day-old infant?

a. bleeding
b. foul odor
c. shriveled, black appearance
d. absence of cord

21-25
B
Appl.
Impl.

The nurse determines that a 48-hour-old infant has not passed meconium. Which nursing intervention has the highest priority at this time?

a. observation of the anal area for fissures
b. digital examination of the anal/rectal area
c. increasing the amount of oral feedings
d. measuring the abdominal girth

21-26
A
Appl.
Impl.

The nurse notes that a newborn sucking on a pacifier responds to noises by briefly ceasing to suck on the pacifier followed by continued sucking. The nurse should respond by:

a. documenting this evidence of normal functioning.
b. immediately evaluating the moro and rooting reflexes.
c. requesting advanced neurological testing.
d. carrying out additional tests to evaluate for possible hearing impairment.

21-27
A
Know.
Asses.

The "blue color" of a neonate's hands and feet is a common and temporary condition called:

a. acrocyanosis.
b. erythema neonatorum.
c. harlequin color.
d. vernix caseosa.

21-28
A
Comp.
Analy.

A small port-wine stain is located on a neonate and pointed out to the parents. Which of the following remarks by the parents would demonstrate no need for further explanation of this mark?

a. "Even though it's permanent, at least it's not too visible."
b. "I hope it goes away soon, so she isn't marked for life."
c. "My grandmother told me not to drink during my pregnancy!"
d. "The doctor must have pulled on her too hard."

21-29
C
Know.
Asses.

The purpose of the rooting reflex in a neonate is:

a. interactive.
b. protective.
c. an aid in feeding.
d. overstimulation defense.

Chapter 22

The Normal Newborn: Needs and Care

Instructions: For each of the following multiple-choice questions, select the ONE most appropriate answer.

22-1
D
Comp.
Impl.

Instillation of medication to prevent opthalmia neonatorum may be deferred in the birthing room primarily so:

    a. routine eye irrigation may be completed.
    b. chances of iatrogenic infection will be reduced.
    c. signs of hypersensitivity will not be overlooked.
    d. eye contact and bonding is facilitated immediately post-delivery.

22-2
C
Appl.
Diag.

An indication that a newborn infant may require additional injections of vitamin K is:

    a. failure to gain weight.
    b. fissures at lip margins.
    c. bleeding from the umbilical cord.
    d. passage of frothy yellow stool.

22-3
A
Appl.
Diag.

Of the following nursing diagnoses relevant to the newborn, which requires the MOST immediate nursing intervention?

    a. Ineffective airway clearance related to mucus obstruction.
    b. Alteration in comfort related to pain of frequent heelsticks.
    c. Alteration in nutrition: less than body requirements related to limited formula intake.
    d. Alteration in urinary elimination related to post-circumcision status.

22-4
C
Know.
Plan.

The PRIMARY purpose of the nursing care plan for the family with a newborn is to:

    a. promote standardized care.
    b. decrease numbers of caregivers relating to the family.
    c. insure that the goals of care are achieved.
    d. speed progression of the family from hospital to home care.

Karen was born by vaginal birth 45 minutes ago. After the initial nursing assessment and parental bonding activities, she is being admitted to the observational nursery.

(THE FOLLOWING 7 ITEMS RELATE TO THE ABOVE PASSAGE.)

22-5
C
Comp.
Impl.

In her/his report of Karen's condition to the nursery staff, the birthing room nurse MUST include:

    a. gestational age assessment.
    b. complete physical exam results.
    c. resuscitative birthing room measures.
    d. observations of parental psychosocial bonding.

22-6   Karen's initial temperature reading should be obtained using the _____ route.
A
Know.   a. axillary
Impl.   b. oral
          c. rectal
          d. skin sensor

22-7   Which of the following nursing interventions is appropriate during Karen's
D   first four hours of life?
Appl.
Impl.   a. bathing her in a tub of warm water
          b. monitoring her temperature every 2 hours
          c. assessing her radial pulse hourly
          d. performing a digital exam to check for rectal patency

22-8   Which of the following is Karen most likely to exhibit during the first period of
A   reactivity?
Comp.
Asses.   a. lack of bowel sounds
          b. no interest in sucking
          c. passage of meconium
          d. decreased arousability from sleep

22-9   Karen's initial nursing care plan lists the goal "maintenance of a clear airway."
A   Which nursing intervention is utilized to meet this goal in a healthy newborn such
Comp.   as Karen?
Impl.
          a. using a DeLee catheter
          b. initiating continuous gastric decompression
          c. vigorous stroking of the abdomen
          d. positioning supine with head slightly elevated

22-10   Initially Karen is placed unclothed under a radiant warmer with a skin sensor
B   attached to her abdomen. The primary reason for placing Karen under the radiant
Comp.   warmer upon admittance to the nursery is to:
Impl.
          a. promote optimal visualization of the infant.
          b. prevent expenditure of energy to maintain homeostasis.
          c. promote drying of the umbilical stump.
          d. allow maximal accessibility to the infant.

22-11   Karen's father is present when she receives her vitamin K injection. He questions
D   why the medication is given in her thigh rather than in her buttock. The nurse's
Appl.   response which provides the best information to the father is:
Impl.
          a. "We never give infants injections in the posterior hip area."
          b. "We use the thigh area because it doesn't have large nerves or major blood
              vessels."
          c. "It is much easier to stabilize Karen's leg when the anterior thigh is used."
          d. "The buttock muscle is not as well developed as the thigh muscles in the
              newborn."

22-12
B
Comp.
Impl.

Following circumcision of the male infant, the nurse should asses the site for signs of hemorrhage and infection and should carefully monitor the urinary output. The nurse should also evaluate the:

a. timing of each voiding.
b. adequacy of the flow of urine.
c. glucose content of the urine.
d. color of the scrotal tissue.

Baby Nick, a 2-day-old, term infant, is of normal weight and length and has had an uncomplicated newborn course while in the birthing center. Nick is his parents' first child.

(THE FOLLOWING 13 ITEMS RELATE TO THE ABOVE PASSAGE.)

22-13
D
Appl.
Impl.

Nick's nurse notes that his parents have wrapped him in three blankets in addition to his clothing. Nick's respiratory rate is higher than normal and he appears restless. Which action by the nurse is most appropriate to meet the goal "maintenance of neutral thermal environment"?

a. Remove Nick from his parents and undress him in the nursery.
b. Undress Nick in the parents' room and take all blankets to the nursery.
c. Undress Nick and place him in a basin of tepid water in the parents' room.
d. Explain Nick's behaviors indicating overheating and remain with Nick's parents as they remove the extra blankets.

22-14
A
Comp.
Impl.

Nick's mother becomes upset when Nick avoids eye contact, turns his head away, and exhibits little movement of his arms and legs when she is playing with him. She states that she is afraid Nick doesn't like her. The nurse's response should be based upon the knowledge that:

a. Nick is exhibiting normal signs of fatigue.
b. poor bonding exists between Nick and his mother.
c. Nick is exhibiting signs of severe illness.
d. Nick needs increased calories to maintain wakefulness.

22-15
C
Appl.
Eval.

Nick's mother is shown various newborn positioning techniques to use with Nick when she takes him home. Which statement by Nick's mother regarding newborn positioning indicates a need for further teaching?

a. "I'll never leave Nick on his back unless I am right there with him."
b. "After I feed Nick, I'll put him on his right side."
c. "If I place Nick on his stomach, he could suffocate."
d. "I'll remember to use different positions so Nick won't get a flat head."

22-16
C
Appl.
Eval.

Which statement by Nick's father demonstrates that he understands the correct technique for nasal/oral suctioning?

a. "I put the bulb in the center of Nick's mouth and slowly release pressure on the bulb."
b. "I put the bulb in Nick's nose, gently squeeze it, and then release it."
c. "I squeeze the bulb first, then put it in Nick's nose or mouth."
d. "I should suction Nick's mouth every time I suction his nose."

22-17
A
Appl.
Eval.

Nick's mother is doing a return demonstration of the sponge bath technique. At which point in the sequential lists of steps below does the nurse need to stop Nick's mother for additional teaching?

a. She tests the tub of soapy water for correct temperature using her elbow.
b. She wipes each of Nick's eyes from inner to outer corner with a separate moistened cotton ball.
c. Each of Nick's external ear areas is washed with the washcloth; no cotton swabs are used.
d. The remainder of Nick's face is washed with the washcloth.

22-18
D
Know.
Eval.

Nick's mother is insistent upon using baby powder on Nick. Which response by the nurse gives the best information concerning the application of powders to newborns?

a. "Sprinkle the powder in the dry diaper and then place the diaper on Nick."
b. "Apply the powder to Nick's body when he is still slightly moist from his bath."
c. "Apply a thin film of baby oil before lightly dusting Nick with a talc-free powder."
d. "The powder should be shaken onto your hands first and then applied to Nick's body."

22-19
C
Appl.
Impl.

The nurse is unable to retract the foreskin on Nick's uncircumcised penis easily as s/he prepares to cleanse his perineal area. At this time s/he should:

a. notify Nick's physician.
b. use force to push the foreskin back.
c. cleanse the exposed area of the glans.
d. use a syringe of soapy water to irrigate under the foreskin.

22-20
A
Appl.
Plan.

Nick's parents express concern about their ability to care for Nick's umbilical cord stump at home. The nurse plans to instruct both parents in proper cord care by having them:

a. cleanse the cord and surrounding skin with alcohol-soaked cotton balls.
b. apply bacitracin ointment to the cord stump several times.
c. watch an instructional filmstrip on newborn hygiene care.
d. read a variety of pamphlets on care of the newborn.

22-21
B
Know.
Impl.

Should Nick develop cradle cap, Nick's parents should be taught to manage it by:

a. applying antibiotic ointment to the scalp after the daily shampoo.
b. moistening the scaly areas with lotion for thirty minutes prior to shampooing.
c. using a firm-bristled brush to scrub the scales off the scalp.
d. washing the hair with gentle shampoo three times daily until the scales disappear.

22-22
D
Comp.
Imp.

Nick's mother expresses concern over Nick's long fingernails. She knows they need to be shortened and questions the nurse concerning the proper technique. The nurse's best response to Nick's mother would be, "You should:

   a. gently bite the excess nail off to avoid injury to Nick's fingers."
   b. clip Nick's fingernails with nailclippers just prior to a feeding."
   c. avoid trimming the nails by allowing them to break off on their own."
   d. trim the nails straight across with cuticle scissors while Nick sleeps."

22-23
D
Know.
Impl.

Nick's parents are taught to take Nick's rectal temperature with Nick positioned:

   a. lying flat on his abdomen.
   b. on his abdomen in a crawling position.
   c. side-lying on his right side with his left leg flexed.
   d. supine with his rectum exposed by holding his legs up in one hand.

22-24
A
Appl.
Eval.

Nick's parents demonstrate good understanding of temperature assessment by stating:

   a. "Nick's temperature needs to be taken only when he shows signs of illness."
   b. "We need to take Nick's axillary temperature every day at home."
   c. "We should only take Nick's rectal temperature at home if he is sick enough to go to the doctor."
   d. "Nick only needs to have his temperature taken when he feels warm to the touch."

22-25
C
Comp.
Eval.

Which of the following statements by Nick's parents demonstrates safe home management practices for the newborn?

   a. "Nick should receive liquid aspirin every three hours if his temperature goes up."
   b. "We should give Nick a small enema if he doesn't have at least 2 stools a day."
   c. "If Nick doesn't wet six diapers a day we need to give him more water."
   d. "We shouldn't allow Nick to sleep more than 12 hours a day."

22-26
D
Know.
Plan.

Current knowledge of the practice of circumcision demonstrates that:

   a. there are few risks of complications.
   b. it promotes optimal health for male infants.
   c. it is essential for adequate male hygienic purposes.
   d. it should be avoided in infants with genitourinary defects.

22-27
A
Comp.
Impl.

For the trip home from the birthing center, the newborn would be adequately protected if transported in:

   a. an approved car seat facing the rear of the car.
   b. the mother's arms while she is seated in the rear of the car.
   c. an infant carrier secured to the rear seat with a seat belt.
   d. an approved car seat facing forward between two passengers in the rear seat.

Chapter 23

Newborn Nutrition

Instructions: For each of the following multiple-choice questions, select the ONE most appropriate answer.

23-1
B
Know.
Diag.

Nutritionally, when compared with a 1-year-old, the newborn requires proportionately:

    a. less vitamin C.
    b. larger amounts of calories and protein.
    c. larger amounts of fat-soluble vitamins.
    d. smaller numbers of total calories from fats and carbohydrates.

23-2
A
Appl.
Impl.

A formula-fed infant with an allergy to milk should not be fed:

    a. Enfamil.
    b. Isomil.
    c. Neomulsoy.
    d. Prosobee.

23-3
D
Appl.
Diag.

The newborn whose urine has a high specific gravity has increased need for:

    a. electrolytes.
    b. minerals.
    c. protein.
    d. water.

23-4
C
Comp.
Diag.

The immature renal system of the newborn would be LEAST taxed by which type of nourishment?

    a. colostrum
    b. mature breast milk
    c. regular infant formula
    d. soy-based formula

23-5
C
Know.
Diag.

In comparison to most prepared formulas, mature breast milk has:

    a. a thicker consistency.
    b. more calories per ounce.
    c. greater immunologic value.
    d. increased proportions of nitrogenous wastes.

23-6
B
Appl.
Impl.

The mother of a newborn states, "I feel so guilty that I was unable to breast-feed my baby." The nurse's response showing the most honesty and support for the mother is:

a. "You did your best. Your baby will not suffer much from the formula."
b. "You really will be able to meet your baby's needs with the formula. Tell me more about your feelings related to your breast-feeding efforts."
c. "Breast-feeding is much better for your baby. Maybe you just didn't try hard enough or long enough to be successful with it."
d. "It's really not your fault. Some babies are just very difficult to breast-feed. They usually end up being picky eaters later in life."

Sara Smith, 3 weeks old, is being breast-fed, appears healthy, and is gaining weight.

(THE FOLLOWING 6 ITEMS RELATE TO THE ABOVE PASSAGE.)

23-7
C
Appl.
Impl.

Mrs. Smith calls the pediatrician's office to report that Sara is not gaining weight as rapidly as her friend's formula-fed baby (born two days prior to Sara). Which of the following would be the best response by the office nurse?

a. "All babies gain weight at a different rate. You shouldn't be making comparisons."
b. "You need to bring Sara in to the office; she may be ill."
c. "Bottle-fed babies do gain weight faster than breast-fed babies, Mrs. Smith. Sara's weight gain is just right for her age."
d. "Your friend is probably overfeeding her baby. She will probably have problems controlling the child's weight in the future."

23-8
D
Appl.
Impl.

Mrs. Smith expresses concern to the pediatrician's office nurse that her friend's formula-fed baby is receiving iron drops. Mrs. Smith wonders if Sara should also receive iron supplementation. Which response by the nurse is based upon current knowledge of iron-supplementation needs of the breast-fed infant?

a. "I'll have the doctor calculate the dosage of iron Sara should receive daily."
b. "For as long as Sara is breast-feeding she won't require iron supplementation."
c. "Sara will not require iron supplements until she reaches three months of age."
d. "If you continue to eat well and take your multivitamins, Sara won't need iron supplements until she is about six months old.

23-9
A
Appl.
Impl.

Mrs. Smith asks, "Is it true that breast milk will prevent Sara from catching colds and other infections?" Which of the following responses is supported by current research?

a. "Sara will have an increased resistance to illness caused by bacteria and viruses, but may still contract infections."
b. "You shouldn't have to worry about Sara's exposure to contagious illness until she stops breast-feeding."
c. "Breast milk offers no greater protection to Sara than formula feedings."
d. "Breast milk will give Sara protection from all illnesses to which you are immune."

23-10
B
Comp.
Eval.

The office nurse questions Mrs. Smith about her feelings during breast-feeding of Sara. This question is an attempt to gather information concerning:

a. feeding technique.
b. maternal attachment.
c. infant behavioral assessment.
d. nutritional adequacy of feedings.

23-11
C
Appl.
Eval.

Which of the following questions by the nurse would generate the MOST information from Mrs. Smith concerning her breast-feeding?

a. "How long does it take for Sara to complete each feeding?"
b. "How often are you feeding Sara each day?"
c. "Tell me how things are going with breast-feeding, Mrs. Smith."
d. "Mrs. Smith, tell me your number one problem with breast-feeding."

23-12
C
Know.
Impl.

Mrs. Smith asks if it will be all right to switch Sara to whole cow's milk if she decides to stop breast-feeding within the next month. The nurses response should be based upon knowledge that whole cow's milk:

a. lacks adequate protein.
b. is an acceptable immediate alternative.
c. should not be used with infants less than 6 months old.
d. may be substituted immediately if Sara receives multivitamins.

23-13
A
Know.
Impl.

The newborn's initial feeding should be:

a. sterile water.
b. glucose water.
c. half-strength formula.
d. warm tap water.

23-14
A
Comp.
Asses.

The nurse would suspect esophageal atresia without fistula in the newborn who takes a formula feeding well initially but regurgitates:

a. unchanged formula.
b. bile-stained formula.
c. blood-tinged formula.
d. curdled, green-stained formula.

23-15
B
Appl.
Impl.

Immediately following birth, a mother asks to breast-feed her newborn. Which of the following nursing interventions is appropriate if the newborn appears healthy?

a. Refuse the request.
b. Assist the mother to attempt breast-feeding.
c. Feed sterile water to evaluate swallowing first.
d. Aspirate stomach contents prior to breast-feeding attempt.

23-16
D
Comp.
Asses.

When comparing the feeding habits of the breast-fed infant to the formula-fed infant, the breast-fed infant:

a. experiences shorter periods between feedings.
b. digests her/his feedings more rapidly.
c. commonly desires to eat every 1 and 1/2 to 3 hours.
d. frequently skips night feedings by age 6 weeks.

23-17
C
Comp.
Impl.

Which situation represents the BEST method for teaching new mothers newborn feeding techniques?

a. Demonstrate a variety of techniques at the initial teaching.
b. Use a number of personnel to insure a wide range of modifications for a single technique.
c. Consistently teach the same procedure for one feeding technique.
d. Teach only broad concepts rather than a specific feeding technique.

Mrs Peterson has chosen to bottle-feed her newborn son. This is Mrs. Peterson's first baby, and she is anxious to learn as much as possible before leaving the birthing center. The staff nurse assigned to Mrs. Peterson has assessed good maternal-infant bonding.

(THE FOLLOWING 5 ITEMS RELATE TO THE ABOVE PASSAGE.)

23-18
B
Appl.
Impl.

The nurse observes that Mrs. Peterson becomes frustrated when she attempts to play with her son immediately following his feeding and he falls asleep. The most helpful intervention by the nurse would be to:

a. remove Mrs. Peterson's son to the nursery immediately after each feeding.
b. initiate playful activity between Mrs. Peterson and her son just prior to his next feeding.
c. remind Mrs. Peterson that her behavior will cause her son to vomit his feedings.
d. give the infant half of his normal feeding prior to taking him to Mrs. Peterson.

23-19
D
Comp.
Eval.

Which behavior by Mrs. Peterson indicates good bottle-feeding technique?

a. props the bottle on a rolled towel
b. points the nipple at the infant's tongue
c. enlarges the nipple hole to allow for a steady stream of formula flow
d. keeps the nipple full of formula throughout the feeding

23-20
C
Appl.
Impl.

Mrs. Peterson attempts to burp her son after every few swallows of formula. He becomes restless and cries, upsetting Mrs. Peterson. Which response by the nurse is most appropriate?

a. "You're burping him much too frequently, Mrs. Peterson."
b. "Just look at how upset your baby has become. Give him to me."
c. "Your burping technique is good, but try burping him only at the middle and end of the feeding."
d. "He's confused, Mrs. Peterson. Put him up on your shoulder to burp him."

23-21
B
Comp.
Impl.

Mrs. Peterson should be taught that when her son regurgitates small amounts of formula, she should:

a. take his rectal temperature.
b. recognize this as a normal occurrence.
c. discontinue feedings for 6 to 8 hours.
d. report this immediately to her pediatrician.

23-22
A
Comp.
Impl.

Mrs. Peterson's son tends to fall asleep before his feeding is completed. Mrs. Peterson should be taught to:

a. use tactile stimulation to arouse sucking.
b. force-feed until the bottle is empty.
c. skip several feedings to increase hunger.
d. increase the size of the nipple opening.

Barbara Johnson recently gave birth to her first child. She successfully began breast-feeding in the birthing room. Her newborn daughter Julie is rooming-in.

(THE FOLLOWING 5 ITEMS RELATE TO THE A ABOVE PASSAGE.)

23-23
C
Comp.
Impl.

Mrs. Johnson experiences strong uterine contractions while feeding Julie. She excitedly rings for the nurse. Upon the nurse's arrival, Mrs Johnson tells her/him, "something must be wrong. I feel like I'm in labor again." Which response by the nurse correctly identifies the physiological response Mrs. Johnson is experiencing?

a. "Your breasts are secreting a hormone that enters your blood stream and causes your abdominal muscles to contract."
b. "Prolactin is speeding the flood supply to your uterus and you are feeling the blood vessel engorgement."
c. "The same hormone which is released in response to Julie's sucking, causing milk flow, also causes the uterus to contract."
d. "You probably have a small blood clot in your uterus which is causing it to contract to expel it."

23-24
D
Know.
Impl.

Of the following nursing interventions, which is a positive intervention for a breast-feeding mother such as Mrs. Johnson?

a. bottle-feeding infants between breast-feedings
b. advocating routine use of nipple shields
c. imposing time limits for breast-feeding sessions
d. encouraging alternating the breast offered first at feedings

23-25
A
Appl.
Eval.

The nurse questions Mrs. Johnson to evaluate her knowledge of storing techniques for expressed milk. Which statement by Mrs. Johnson indicates a need for additional teaching?

a. "I'll boil the milk just prior to feeding it to Julie."
b. "After expressing the milk, I'll need to freeze it."
c. "I'll need to make sure that I have plastic bottles for storing the milk."
d. "The wrong type of bottle will decrease the breast milk's protective function."

23-26
B
Appl.
Eval.

Which action by Mrs. Johnson indicates an understanding of the potential effects of maternal medications on Julie? Mrs. Johnson:

a. requests pain medication 30 minutes prior to breast-feeding Julie.
b. reminds her obstetrician that she is breast-feeding when s/he hands her 3 discharge prescriptions.
c. reminds her husband to bring her time-released hay fever medication from home.
d. refuses decaffeinated coffee stating, "I need at least four cups of regular coffee to get me moving every morning."

23-27
C
Comp.
Impl.

Which action by Mrs. Johnson is contraindicated to decrease breast engorgement?

a. nursing Julie more frequently
b. wearing a nursing bra 24 hours a day
c. applying ice packs just prior to feeding Julie
d. utilizing a warm shower for comfort

23-28
C
Comp.
Impl.

A young mother calls the nurse to report feeding problems she is experiencing with her 3-month-old son. "Every time I put the spoon in his mouth he spits the food back at me." Which response by the nurse is based upon sound knowledge of infant nutrition and infant behavior?

a. "Rice cereal would be easier for him to swallow."
b. "Have you tried fruits or other sweet-tasting foods?"
c. "Because he is not developmentally ready for solid foods, a tongue thrusting reflex causes him to push the food out of his mouth."
d. "Blenderize fresh vegetables or fresh fruits without adding salt or sugar and offer these prior to his formula."

Chapter 24

The Newborn at Risk

Instructions: For each of the following multiple-choice questions, select the ONE most appropriate answer.

24-1
D
Comp.
Asses.

In assessing the newborn for at-risk status, it is now known that:

a. any infant with a birth weight of less than 2,500 grams is preterm.
b. the large-for-gestational-age infant has little risk of neonatal morbidity.
c. gestational age is the one criterion utilized to establish mortality risk.
d. infants who are preterm and small for gestational age have the highest mortality risk.

24-2
D
Know.
Plan.

Nursing diagnoses relevant to the birth of an at-risk newborn must focus upon the:

a. newborn alone.
b. newborn and the mother.
c. newborn, father, and mother.
d. newborn and all family members affected by this birth.

24-3
C
Appl.
Diag.

Which of the following assessments represents the MOST important determining factor for development of respiratory distress in the preterm neonate?

a. acidemia
b. Apgar 5 at 5 minutes
c. alveolar collapse with exhalation
d. meconium staining on skin

Alex is a preterm infant born at 34 weeks' gestation. He is two days old and his weight is average for gestational age (AGA).

(THE FOLLOWING 9 ITEMS RELATE TO THE ABOVE PASSAGE.)

24-4
B
Comp.
Plan.

The nurse is very concerned about Alex's ability to maintain a normal body temperature. S/he is aware that Alex has limited heat production capabilities as exhibited by his:

a. extended posture.
b. small muscle mass.
c. proximity of blood vessels to skin surface.
d. limited amount of subcutaneous fat.

24-5
A
Comp.
Plan.

The nurse is aware that Alex's nutritional status is compromised by the expected preterm gastrointestinal problem of:

a. abnormal protein metabolism.
b. increased absorption of fats.
c. simple sugar malabsorption.
d. malformed gastrointestinal tract structures.

24-6
B
Appl.
Impl.

Because of Alex's immature neurologic system, the nurse must closely monitor for signs of:

a. malabsorption.
b. aspiration.
c. infection.
d. anemia.

24-7
A
Comp.
Impl.

Because Alex has immature liver functioning, the nurse must carefully monitor:

a. blood glucose.
b. serum amylase.
c. blood urea nitrogen.
d. white blood cell count.

24-8
D
Appl.
Plan.

The nurse carefully evaluates Alex's behavioral sleep-wake states. S/he utilizes information gained from this assessment process when s/he:

a. selects lab tests.
b. schedules medication administration.
c. calculates fluid administration rates.
d. determines the parental visitation schedule.

24-9
C
Know.
Impl.

Most formulas for preterm infants such as Alex contain _____ calories per ounce.

a. 16
b. 20
c. 24
d. 28

24-10
D
Appl.
Eval.

Alex is carefully monitored prior to the initiation of nipple-feeding. In which of the following situations would nipple-feeding be contraindicated?

a. gaining weight; coordinated suck-swallow reflex
b. alert; axillary temperature of 97 degrees F
c. apical heart rate 120; skin temperature of 36.5 degrees C
d. nasal flaring; sustained respiratory rate of 68

24-11
B
Comp.
Eval.

Indications that Alex is within normal limits for fluid and nutritional status are:

a. blood pH of 7.25 and urine specific gravity of 1.000.
b. negative dipstix and dextrostix value of 90.
c. tremulousness and dextrostix less than 45 mg/dL.
d. urine specific gravity 1.025, positive clinitest.

24-12
C
Appl.
Impl.

Alex experiences an apneic spell which is nonresponsive to tactile stimulation. His heart rate is bradycardic and he is dusky. The nurse's first intervention should be:

a. give 100% O_2 by mask.
b. prepare for intubation.
c. suction naso- and oropharynx.
d. initiate cardiopulmonary resuscitation.

24-13
D
Comp.
Diag.

Like the preterm infant, the newborn with postmaturity syndrome is at high risk for cold stress due to:

a. extended posture.
b. absence of vernix.
c. parchment-like skin.
d. decreased subcutaneous tissue.

24-14
D
Know.
Asses.

In order for a newborn to be classified as small for gestational age, s/he must:

a. weigh less than 2500 grams.
b. be born prior to the 38th week of gestation.
c. have suffered growth retardation secondary to placental malfunction.
d. be at or below the 10th percentile on a gestational age/birth weight chart.

24-15
C
Appl.
Diag.

Early provision of enteral or parenteral glucose is of primary importance in the small for gestational age (SGA) newborn to:

a. promote weight gain.
b. promote glycogen storage.
c. protect CNS function.
d. accelerate body fat deposition.

Christina is the newborn infant of a class B (White's Scale) diabetic mother. She is 25 minutes old and has been taken to the nursery for close observation.

(THE FOLLOWING 3 ITEMS RELATE TO THE ABOVE PASSAGE.)

24-16
B
Comp.
Plan.

The primary nurse should anticipate that medical management of Christina's hyperinsulinism will involve:

a. insulin-blocker drugs.
b. hydration with 10-15% intravenous glucose solution.
c. transfusion with packed red blood cells.
d. intravenous infusion of supplemental calcium solution.

24-17
D
Comp.
Diag.

In comparison to infants of diabetic mothers suffering poor uterine blood supply, Christina is at higher risk for developing:

a. hypocalcemia.
b. polycythemia.
c. hyperbilirubinemia.
d. respiratory distress.

24-18
B
Appl.
Diag.

Christina's mother states that she finds it difficult to believe that Christina may have problems because she looks so "pink and chubby." The nurse's response to Christina's mother should be based upon knowledge that these signs are physiologic manifestations of:

a. edema and acidosis.
b. increased body fat and polycythemia.
c. gluconeogenesis and hyperbilirubinemia.
d. muscle hypertrophy and hypocalcemia.

24-19
A
Know.
Plan.

The most common and serious problem associated with fetal alcohol syndrome is:

a. CNS dysfunction.
b. midface malformation.
c. immune deficiency.
d. growth deficiency.

24-20
A
Know.
Impl.

Which of the following is contraindicated in treatment of the narcotic-addicted pregnant woman?

a. complete narcotic withdrawal
b. nutritional assessment and modification
c. replacement of heroin use with methadone
d. pharmacologic management of existing infections

24-21
A
Appl.
Impl.

In the neonate experiencing neonatal withdrawal, nursing interventions for the nursing diagnosis "alteration in skin integrity related to hyperactive movements" include:

a. swaddling.
b. positioning on right side.
c. feeding with 24 calorie/oz. formula.
d. maintenance of thermoneutral environment.

24-22
D
Appl.
Asses.

An infant is born with a major facial anomaly. Which of the following maternal comments is most characteristic of the parental adjustment phase of depression?

a. "I just keep forgetting that this has happened."
b. "How many other babies were born that day? You must have gotten them confused."
c. "I've talked with the surgeon. It's going to take a long time, but we'll make it happen."
d. "Why did God do this to me? He's given me so much more than I'll be able to handle."

24-23
D
Comp.
Impl.

A high-risk neonate requires immediate transfer to a distant intensive care nursery. Which nursing action is MOST facilitative of parental attachment? The nurse should provide the parents with:

a. a daily phone report of the neonate's health status.
b. a visit from a transport team member after the transport.
c. verbal explanations of the neonate's treatment plan.
d. photographs of the neonate.

24-24
A
Comp.
Asses.

Physiologic adaption is a greater stressor for premature infants than for full-term infants because premature infants' body systems are not fully developed. In the premature infant the nurse would expect to see:

a. jaundice.
b. hyperglycemia.
c. birth trauma.
d. aspiration of meconium.

24-25
B
Appl.
Plan.

Baby Johnson, a 1250 g premature infant, requires 120 to 150 calories/kilogram/day for growth. This means he will need _____ calories per day.

a. 125 to 160
b. 150 to 188
c. 175 to 225
d. 1500 to 1875

24-26
C
Appl.
Plan.

To provide formula for baby Johnson, the nurse has the choice of 3 calorie concentrations: 13 calories/ounce; 20 calories/ounce; or 24 calories/ounce. Which of these would be best, and why?

a. 13 calories/ounce, because it provides extra fluid.
b. 20 calories/ounce, because it provides both fluid and calories.
c. 24 calories/ounce, because it provides greater calories in less volume.
d. none of these, because baby Johnson is too young to be receiving any formula.

Mrs. Walker is admitted to the hospital for delivery. She has a previous obstetric history of fetal death at eight months gestation of undetermined cause. Because of her history, fetal biophysical and biochemical monitoring is planned during the intrapartal period.

(THE FOLLOWING 3 ITEMS RELATE TO THE ABOVE PASSAGE.)

24-27
C
Appl.
Impl.

During active labor, a fetal scalp blood sample with a pH of 7.22 is obtained. Which initial action by the labor and delivery team is most appropriate at this time?

a. Deliver the fetus immediately.
b. Obtain serial fetal pH readings for comparison.
c. Check maternal venous pH and fetal heart rate pattern.
d. Increase the rate of the maternal IV infusion and apply an oxygen mask.

24-28
B
Appl.
Impl.

Baby boy Walker is born. Which action by the nurse is the appropriate initial newborn resuscitation step?

a. inserting a nasogastric tube
b. suctioning the oro- and nasopharynx
c. inflating the lungs with positive pressure
d. positioning the head in the "sniffling position"

24-29
B
Appl.
Impl.

Baby boy Walker begins spontaneous respirations. Which action by the nurse now has priority?

a. Insert an umbilical vein catheter.
b. Dry him quickly under a radiant warmer.
c. Apply continued tactile stimulation to his back.
d. Prepare sodium bicarbonate and epinephrine solutions.

Larry is a black, preterm, male infant born to a class B diabetic mother. He suffered a period of asphyxia during birth but responded to suctioning and oxygen delivery. He was taken to the hospital's high-risk nursery for management.

(THE FOLLOWING 3 ITEMS RELATE TO THE ABOVE PASSAGE.)

24-30   Which of the following manifestations is consistent with a diagnosis for Larry of
A   RDS?
Comp.
Asses.   a. grunting respirations
            b. decreasing respiratory rate
            c. increasing serum pH
            d. decreasing pCO_2 levels

24-31   Larry's clinical course declines and he is classified as experiencing severe RDS.
C   The nurse notifies the cardiopulmonary therapists to set up a/an:
Comp.
Plan.   a. ventimask.
            b. oxyhood.
            c. mechanical ventilator.
            d. low-flow nasal cannula.

24-32   An important intervention for Larry's nursing diagnosis of "ineffective airway
C   clearance related to increased secretions" is:
Comp.
Impl.   a. monitor O_2 concentration every hour.
            b. secure and maintain endotracheal tube with tape.
            c. check proper functioning of suction machine every shift.
            d. observe for evidence of spontaneous respiratory effort.

24-33   During birth, the nurse observes that there is meconium staining of the amniotic
B   fluid and slow, irregular fetal heart rate. The nurse should IMMEDIATELY:
Appl.
Impl.   a. increase rate of the maternal IV.
            b. report her/his observations to the delivering physician.
            c. stimulate the newborn after birth to increase respiratory effort.
            d. bag with O_2 after the head is born.

24-34   Presence of meconium in the lungs:
D
Know.   a. prevents air leaks.
Asses.   b. leads to respiratory alkalosis.
            c. prevents air from entering the airways.
            d. traps inspired air in the alveoli.

24-35   A small gestational age (SGA) neonate has experienced cold stress. Of the
B   following nursing actions, which is CONTRAINDICATED in the care of this
Comp.   neonate?
Impl.
            a. Monitor skin temperature every 15 minutes.
            b. Institute measures for rapid temperature elevation.
            c. Initiate dextrostix monitoring of blood glucose levels.
            d. Observe for clinical manifestations of metabolic acidosis.

        Angela is a neonate who experienced symptomatic hypoglycemia and required an
        intravenous infusion of dextrose. Her condition has stabilized and the physician has
        changed her to oral feedings.

        (THE FOLLOWING 2 ITEMS RELATE TO THE ABOVE PASSAGE.)

24-36
D
Appl.
Impl.

As Angela begins oral feedings the nurse should anticipate that medical orders will include:

   a. discontinuing of IV after first formula feeding.
   b. administering long-acting epinephrine.
   c. giving a bolus intravenous infusion of 25% dextrose.
   d. reinstituting frequent glucose monitoring during the transition.

24-37
B
Comp.
Impl.

In addition to assessment for manifestation of hypoglycemia, Angela's nurse must intervene to conserve Angela's energy stores by:

   a. discontinuing heelsticks.
   b. decreasing crying episodes.
   c. lowering the environmental temperature.
   d. preventing nonnutritive sucking efforts.

24-38
B
Know.
Diag.

The MAJOR concern for the neonate with a high concentration of unconjugated bilirubin is:

   a. jaundice.
   b. neurotoxicity.
   c. liver damage.
   d. renal malfunction.

24-39
B
Know.
Diag.

The parents of a newborn receiving phototherapy request information on how the treatment lowers serum bilirubin levels. The nurse's best response is based on the knowledge that phototherapy:

   a. reverses the causative factors of hyperbilirubinemia.
   b. facilitates excretion of unconjugated bilirubin.
   c. blocks movement of bilirubin from tissues to the blood.
   d. reduces the rate of red blood cell hemolysis.

24-40
D
Appl.
Impl.

A neonate undergoing phototherapy experiences increased urine output and loose stools. The nurse should:

   a. institute enteric isolation.
   b. immediately discontinue phototherapy.
   c. decrease the phototherapy unit's level of irradiance.
   d. observe for clinical manifestations of dehydration.

Ted Mead, a 2-day-old term neonate, has a congenital cardiac malformation with resultant cyanosis. His mother, Susie Mead, is a single parent.

24-41
A
Comp.
Diag.

Ted's cyanosis is directly related to the:

   a. blood flow dynamics.
   b. size of the malformation.
   c. location of the malformation.
   d. total functional alveolar surface area.

24-42
C
Know.
Eval.

The laboratory evaluation for diagnosis of sepsis neonatorum always includes cultures of:

a. rectal secretions.
b. gastric secretions.
c. spinal fluid.
d. nasopharyngeal secretions.

24-43
C
Appl.
Impl.

In teaching parents about dietary management of a child with phenylketonuria, the nurse should emphasize the importance of:

a. discontinuing the special diet when the child reaches 6 years of age.
b. maintaining the special diet until the physician has stated myelination is complete.
c. reinstating the special diet of the female with PKU throughout pregnancy.
d. limiting all nutritional intakes to the low phenylalanine formula throughout the specified time of the diet.

PART 5

POSTPARTUM

Chapter 25

Postpartal Adaptation and Nursing Assessment

Instructions: For each of the following multiple-choice questions, select the ONE most appropriate answer.

Lisa Gill, gravida 1 para 1, vaginally delivered a 7-pound baby girl at 4 p.m. It is now 4:30 p.m. and Lisa has just been admitted to the postpartum unit.

(THE FOLLOWING 6 ITEMS RELATE TO THE ABOVE PASSAGE.)

25-1
D
Know.
Asses.

When assessing the level of Lisa's uterus, the nurse would expect the fundus to be located :

a. at the umbilicus.
b. at the symphysis pubis.
c. midway between the umbilicus and the xiphoid process.
d. midway between the umbilicus and the symphysis pubis.

25-2
B
Appl.
Impl.

During the assessment the nurse notices Lisa's uterus is firm, no clots are expressed, and there is a continuous flow of vaginal blood. In regard to these findings the nurse should:

a. reassure Lisa that this is normal.
b. notify the physician or midwife.
c. apply an ice pack to the perineum.
d. massage the uterus every 15 minutes.

25-3
D
Comp.
Impl.

During her first postpartum day, Lisa asks the nurse how long the vaginal discharge will last. The nurse's best reply would be, "The discharge will last:

a. two to 3 days."
b. about 6 weeks."
c. until the uterine lining has sloughed off."
d. until the placental site has healed."

25-4
A
Comp.
Asses.

Lisa's vaginal discharge is dark red and contains shreds of the decidua and epithelial cells. The nurse should describe the discharge in her nurse's notes as:

a. rubra.
b. serosa.
c. alba.
d. erythra.

25-5
A
Appl.
Impl.

On the day of her delivery Lisa is assisted out of bed for the first time. She becomes frightened when she passes a blood clot and notices an increase in her lochia. The nurse should explain to Lisa that:

a. the lochia pools in the vagina when lying in bed.
b. placental fragments have probably been retained in the uterus.
c. she probably has a uterine or urinary tract infection.
d. the amount of lochia will increase during the postpartum period.

25-6
B
Comp.
Impl.

Lisa asks the nurse when she will start to menstruate again. The nurse should tell Lisa that her menstrual period will begin:

a. in 4 weeks.
b. in 6 to 24 weeks.
c. when ovulation resumes.
d. when the placental site has healed.

Mrs. Martha Jones recently underwent vaginal delivery of her second daughter. She is breast-feeding her new infant without difficulty.

(THE FOLLOWING 5 ITEMS RELATE TO THE ABOVE PASSAGE.)

25-7
B
Appl.
Asses.

On the second day postpartum, the nurse assesses Martha's uterus and finds it located 4 cm below the umbilicus. The nurse would expect this finding to be a result of:

a. bedrest.
b. breast-feeding.
c. retained placental fragments.
d. overdistention of the uterus.

25-8
C
Appl.
Impl.

Martha asks the nurse when the red stretch marks on her abdomen and breast will disappear. The nurse's best response would be, "The stretch marks:

a. will disappear in approximately 6 weeks."
b. are a result of pregnancy and will not disappear."
c. will eventually fade to silver or white."
d. will disappear with the use of vitamin E oil."

25-9
D
Appl.
Impl.

During her discharge teaching, Martha asks the nurse what exercises she can do to prevent female problems in the future. The nurse should encourage Martha to:

a. do modified sit-ups at least 3 times a day.
b. wear a supportive girdle during the day.
c. contract the pelvic before lifting heavy objects.
d. contract and relax the perineum frequently.

25-10
B
Comp.
Diag.

10 days after delivery, Martha returns to the out-patient clinic to be checked by the midwife. The midwife determines that Martha's uterus is located 1 cm above the the symphysis pubis. This is MOST likely an indication of:

a. involution.
b. subinvolution.
c. a response to lactation.
d. a full bladder.

25-11
B
Know.
Asses.

During Martha's vaginal examination, the midwife looks for the return of the vaginal rugae. The rugae will begin to return in approximately:

a. 1 week.
b. 3 weeks.
c. 4 weeks.
d. 6 weeks.

Mrs. Cindy Jackson, para 1 gravida 1, vaginally delivered a term baby a few minutes ago. She seems to be apprehensive and uncertain what to expect during her postpartum convalescence.

(THE FOLLOWING 6 ITEMS RELATE TO THE ABOVE PASSAGE.)

25-12
C
Appl.
Impl.

Immediately after delivery Cindy begins to shake uncontrollably. The nurse should do which of the following?

a. Notify the physician or midwife.
b. Take her temperature in 30 minutes.
c. Cover her with a warm blanket.
d. Encourage her to take slow deep breaths.

25-13
D
Comp.
Asses.

Cindy's vital signs are: temperature 99 degrees F, pulse 80, respirations 16, and blood pressure 134/88. Which one of Cindy's vital signs should the nurse be concerned about?

a. pulse 80
b. respirations 16
c. temperature 99 degrees F
d. blood pressure 134/88

25-14
A
Comp.
Impl.

Because of the soreness in her perineum, Cindy states that she is afraid to have a bowel movement. The nurse should encourage Cindy to:

a. ambulate frequently, eat fresh fruits and vegetables, and drink 6 to 8 glasses of water per day.
b. ask her physician to prescribe a laxative to stimulate defecation.
c. drink 2 glasses of warm water after every meal, then try to defecate.
d. do Kegel exercises twice a day, eat a low roughage diet, and drink 10 glasses of water per day.

25-15
B
Comp.
Asses.

During the second postpartal day, the nurse notices Cindy is talkative but seems to be hesitant about making decisions. The nurse should understand that according to Rubin, Cindy is:

a. having trouble bonding with the infant.
b. in the "taking in" phase.
c. in the "taking hold" phase.
d. experiencing postpartum depression.

25-16
C
Know.
Asses.

Psychologically, at this time Cindy is probably MOST concerned about:

a. getting adequate rest.
b. caring for the new baby.
c. changes in her appearance.
d. changes in her lifestyle.

25-17
A
Know.
Asses.

The process that a mother uses to learn mothering behavior and become comfortable with her identity as a mother is known as:

a. maternal role attainment.
b. maternal bonding.
c. role identity development.
d. self-concept development.

Mrs. Jill Peterson delivered her third baby vaginally yesterday. She is breast-feeding the baby without difficulty.

(THE FOLLOWING 6 ITEMS RELATE TO THE ABOVE PASSAGE.)

25-18
A
Appl.
Asses.

When the nurse palpates Jill's uterus, s/he assesses that it is 2 cm above the umbilicus and located on the left side of the abdomen. The nurse should suspect that Jill probably has:

a. a full bladder.
b. subinvolution.
c. normal involution.
d. an infection.

25-19
B
Appl.
Diag.

When assessing Jill's breasts, the nurse notices a generalized swelling in the upper outer quadrant of the right breast. Jill asks the nurse what could be causing the swelling. The nurse's best response would be, "The swelling is most likely caused by:

a. a localized site of infection."
b. a blockage of one of the milk ducts."
c. a harmless fatty tumor."
d. an enlarged lymph node."

25-20 When the nurse enters Jill's room to perform a postpartum assessment, Jill complains
A   that she is having severe afterbirth pains. The nurse should:
Appl.
Impl. a. medicate Jill for the pain and delay the assessment.
       b. perform the assessment to determine the cause of the alleged pain.
       c. have Jill ambulate to contract the uterus.
       d. massage the uterus to expel any retained blood clots.

25-21 Jill would be suspected of having an infection if which of the following temperature
D   patterns were noted? A temperature:
Know.
Asses. a. above 99 degrees F that persists for any 2 days during the postpartal period.
       b. of 101 degrees F during the first 24 hours after delivery.
       c. above 100.4 degrees F that occurs anytime during the postpartal period.
       d. of 100.4 degrees F or above on any 2 of the first 10 postpartal days.

25-22 Many cultural practices related to childbirth are concerned with:
A
Know. a. consumption of specific foods and avoidance of cold foods.
Asses. b. caring for the infant's umbilical site.
       c. anointing the mother with special herbs.
       d. keeping the infant in close contact with the mother.

25-23 According to Rubin, postpartum depression occurs on which postpartum days?
B
Know. a. first, second and third
Asses. b. third, fifth and seventh
       c. fourth, fifth and sixth
       d. seventh, ninth and tenth

       Mrs. Randi Clark, para 1 gravida 1, delivered a baby boy by cesarean birth. She
       has a bandage over a vertical, abdominal incision and has decided to try breast-
       feeding the baby.

       (THE FOLLOWING 4 ITEMS RELATE TO THE ABOVE PASSAGE.)

25-24 When assessing the firmness and position of Randi's uterus, the nurse should
C   gently palpate:
Know.
Asses. a. above the incision.
       b. below the incision.
       c. on each side of the incision.
       d. through the incision.

25-25 When assessing the uterus, the nurse determines that Randi has uterine atony. The
C   nurse should have Randi do which of the following?
Appl.
Impl. a. ambulate in the hall
       b. perform Kegel exercises
       c. nurse the baby
       d. massage the uterus

25-26
D
Comp.
Impl.

To check for inverted nipples, the nurse will instruct Randi to:

a. rub the nipples vigorously with a terry towel.
b. massage anhydrous lanolin into the nipples and areola.
c. push the nipples inward toward the chest.
d. pull the nipples outward away from the chest.

25-27
B
Appl.
Impl.

Randi complains that she has severe abdominal cramps whenever she nurses the baby. The nurse should explain that:

a. the sympathetic nervous system is stimulated when the baby nurses.
b. oxytocin which causes the uterus to contract is released when the baby sucks.
c. the cramps will decrease if she will massage the uterus before nursing the baby.
d. the cramps will stop when all of the blood clots have been expelled from the uterus.

Mrs. Rebecca Smith vaginally delivered a 7-pound, term, baby boy earlier today.

(THE FOLLOWING 4 ITEMS RELATE TO THE ABOVE PASSAGE.)

25-28
C
Comp.
Asses.

During a routine assessment, the nurse notices Rebecca's vaginal discharge is pink and measures approximately 4 inches on the perineal pad. As the nurse documents her/his assessment data in the woman's chart, which of the following would be the best description of this finding?

a. lochia: moderate/alba
b. lochia: small/rubra
c. lochia: moderate/serosa
d. lochia: scant/blanca

25-29
B
Appl.
Impl.

Rebecca informed the nurse that she passed a blood clot when she voided. The best response by the nurse would be to tell Rebecca to:

a. inform her physician the next time s/he visits.
b. save all future clots expelled.
c. expect numerous clots to be expelled.
d. massage her fundus after expelling a clot.

25-30
B
Know.
Asses.

During the normal postpartal period, the nurse would expect Rebecca to use approximately _____ perineal pads per day.

a. 4
b. 6
c. 10
d. 12

25-31
C
Comp.
Asses.

In order to assess for diastasis recti, the nurse will instruct and/or assist Rebecca in:

a. performing the "pelvic tilt."
b. contracting her buttocks.
c. raising her head from the bed.
d. relaxing her abdominal muscles.

25-32
A
Comp.
Asses.

When Candy's baby was first born, she touched the baby's arms and legs with her fingertips. The nurse should recognize this as:

a. normal mother-infant interaction.
b. maternal fear and uncertainty.
c. maternal embarrassment and discomfort.
d. probable difficulty with bonding.

Janet and Phil Butler delivered their first baby in a birthing center. After birth the family has remained together constantly.

(THE FOLLOWING 4 ITEMS RELATE TO THE ABOVE PASSAGE.)

25-33
C
Appl.
Plan

Which statement by the nurse would help Janet and Phil bond with their baby?

a. "The baby is so quiet in the nursery; he will probably be a perfect baby at home."
b. "Have the grandparents seen the baby yet?"
c. "The baby's eyes look like his father's."
d. "The hospital photographer will be around tomorrow to take pictures."

25-34
D
Appl.
Impl.

Janet is concerned that she doesn't believe the baby has really been born and that she doesn't feel close to it yet. The nurse should tell her that:

a. she would be glad to have the social worker come and see her.
b. research has shown that when the father is present at the birth the maternal feelings are delayed.
c. maternal feelings are usually not present at the birth of the first baby.
d. these feelings are normal and will change with time.

25-35
B
Appl.
Asses.

Which of the following behaviors would indicate that Janet was bonding with her baby?

a. Janet asks her husband to give the baby a bottle of water.
b. Janet talks to the baby and picks him up when he cries.
c. Janet feeds the baby every 3 hours.
d. Janet asks the nurse to recommend a good child care manual.

25-36
A
Appl.
Asses.

It is important for the nurse to assess how the mother felt about the baby before it was born because:

a. the feelings the mother had during pregnancy will affect her relationship with the baby.
b. often the mother will be able to sense if the baby has an abnormality.
c. the feelings indicate whether the baby's and mother's schedules are compatible.
d. the nurse will be able to determine if reality matches the mother's expectations.

Chapter 26

The Postpartal Family: Needs and Care

Instructions: For each of the following multiple-choice questions, select the ONE most appropriate answer.

Linda Wills vaginally delivered a 6-pound baby girl 10 hours ago. She is fidgeting and states her bottom feels like it is tight and on fire. Her vital signs are stable and she does not seem to be in extreme distress.

(THE FOLLOWING 7 ITEMS RELATE TO THE ABOVE PASSAGE.)

26-1
B
Appl.
Asses.

Which of the following diagnoses would have priority for Linda?

a. knowledge deficit
b. alteration in comfort
c. alteration in elimination; constipation
d. alteration in parenting

26-2
A
Know.
Plan.

To promote the comfort and healing of the episiotomy, what is often applied immediately after birth?

a. ice pack
b. heat lamp
c. topical anesthetic
d. antibiotic ointment

26-3
A
Appl.
Impl.

To help Linda sit more comfortably, the nurse should encourage her to:

a. contract her buttocks before sitting or rising.
b. support her weight on the arms of the chair when moving.
c. use a straight-back chair to sit in.
d. sit on an inflatable ring.

26-4
B
Comp.
Asses.

The mother's pain threshold is influenced by all of the following EXCEPT:

a. level of fatigue.
b. cultural background.
c. feelings about the infant.
d. prior experiences.

26-5
A
Comp.
Asses.

On the first postpartal day, Linda wants to talk about the labor and delivery experience. This activity is important for the mother in order to:

a. establish the reality of the experience.
b. prevent social isolation.
c. develop maternal role model behavior.
d. adjust to the loss of her independence.

26-6 Linda tells the nurse that she doesn't understand why she doesn't feel like the baby
C   is really hers. She thought that having a baby would be wonderful. To help Linda
Appl. express her feelings the nurse should:
Impl.

    a. assure Linda that most new mothers feel unsure about caring for a new baby.
    b. tell Linda that as she begins to care for the baby, she will love the baby.
    c. ask Linda to describe what she thought having a baby was going to be like.
    d. relate how she felt when she had her first baby and that she was able to cope.

26-7 In order to assess how Linda is bonding with the infant, the nurse should:
B
Appl.   a. ask Linda if she is having any difficulty in caring for the baby.
Asses.   b. observe Linda feeding the baby and watch her reactions when the baby cries.
    c. ask Linda's husband if Linda is able to care for the baby without help.
    d. determine if Linda has been to child care classes or has read any books.

Mrs. Collins has just delivered her first baby by cesarean birth. This is her first
postoperative day.

(THE FOLLOWING 7 ITEMS RELATE TO THE ABOVE PASSAGE.)

26-8 Mrs. Collins asked the nurse why she has to cough, turn and deep breathe when
B   it causes her incision to hurt so much. The nurse should tell her that:
Appl.
Impl.   a. she needs to blow off the anesthetic she received during surgery.
    b. she needs to fully inflate her lungs to prevent the pooling of secretions.
    c. the physician has ordered the exercise for her to help her recover faster.
    d. the breathing, turning and coughing will decrease the amount of pain
       medication she will require.

26-9 Mrs. Collins complains that her back and shoulders are sore. The nurse should
D   first:
Appl.
Impl.   a. give her the analgesic that has been ordered.
    b. assess the incisional site and amount of lochia.
    c. take her vital signs and call the physician.
    d. give her a back rub and change her position.

26-10 The nurse tells Mrs. Collins that she should not drink cokes, use a straw, or eat
A   sweets. Mrs. Collins asks the nurse why she has these restrictions. The nurse
Appl. should tell her that:
Impl.
    a. these practices tend to increase gas for some mothers.
    b. since she is nursing, these practices are not good for the baby.
    c. her intestines will be sluggish for a few days and absorption will be
       decreased.
    d. these restrictions are necessary to prevent nausea.

26-11   When the nurse helps Mrs. Collins nurse her baby, the nurse should suggest that
B   Mrs. Collins:
Appl.
Impl.   a. place a pillow on her abdomen to cushion the infant.
         b. lie on her side to nurse the baby.
         c. wash her nipples with soap and water first.
         d. give the baby glucose water following the feeding.

26-12   When teaching Mrs. Collins how to do leg exercises, the nurse should have Mrs.
D   Collins:
Appl.
Impl.   a. raise and lower each leg alternately.
         b. raise both legs off the bed and hold for 5 seconds.
         c. bend the knee, lift the leg, then straighten the knee 10 times for each leg.
         d. bend and straighten the knee, and dorsiflex and plantarflex the foot.

26-13   How often should Mrs. Collins do leg exercises during the day of birth?
B
Know.   a. every 15 minutes
Plan.   b. every 2 hours
         c. 3 times per day
         d. 2 times per day

26-14   When helping Mrs. Collins get out of a bed that does not move and that does not have
C   side rails, the nurse should have Mrs. Collins:
Appl.
Impl.   a. sit up in bed for a few minutes before walking.
         b. reach up to the headboard to pull herself out of bed.
         c. turn to the side and use her arms to raise her upper body from the bed.
         d. turn to the side and then get on her hands and knees before getting out of bed.

Jill Jones, 15 years old, has just delivered her first child vaginally. She had no
prenatal care and her knowledge about care of herself and the baby is limited.

(THE FOLLOWING 6 ITEMS RELATE TO THE ABOVE PASSAGE.)

26-15   Which of the following nursing diagnoses would have priority for Jill?
D
Appl.   a. potential fluid volume deficit
Asses.   b. alteration in nutrition; less than body requirements
         c. alteration in comfort; pain
         d. knowledge deficit

26-16   In order to act as a role model for Jill, the nurse should:
A
Appl.   a. cuddle and talk to the infant.
Impl.   b. take the baby to the nursery when it cries.
         c. tell Jill how to give the baby a bottle.
         d. help Jill plan for the future with the baby.

149

26-17
D
Appl.
Plan.

When the nurse is planning to teach Jill about postpartum care for herself and care of the baby, the nurse would expect that Jill would benefit MOST from:

a. individual instruction.
b. group lectures.
c. pamphlets developed by the hospital.
d. group discussion with peers.

26-18
A
Appl.
Impl.

Jill tells the nurse that having the baby is going to be wonderful. Which response by the nurse would evaluate the accuracy of Jill's beliefs?

a. "Tell me what your day will be like when you take the baby home."
b. "Will anyone be available to help you at home with the baby?"
c. "Have you ever had any experience taking care of young children?"
d. "What are you going to do with the baby while you are in school or working?"

26-19
B
Comp.
Plan.

Prior to discharge Jill has learned to physically care for her baby. In order to promote normal growth and development, the nurse should stress:

a. adequate infant weight gain.
b. infant stimulation.
c. prevention of infection.
d. assumption of maternal role.

26-20
C
Comp.
Impl.

In order to provide Jill with help at home the nurse should:

a. arrange for a nurse to stay with Jill.
b. schedule a well-baby check-up for Jill.
c. give Jill the telephone numbers of the nursery postpartum unit.
d. tell Jill to ask her mother any questions she has.

Mrs. Hill delivered her second daughter vaginally early this morning.

(THE FOLLOWING 4 ITEMS RELATE TO THE ABOVE PASSAGE.)

26-21
C
Appl.
Impl.

To promote comfort during breast-feeding the nurse should:

a. massage the fundus before the baby nurses.
b. have the mother use a nipple shield when the baby nurses.
c. administer an analgesic one hour before the baby will nurse.
d. have Mrs. Hill perform Kegel exercises while she nurses the baby.

26-22
C
Comp.
Plan.

Mrs. Hill is getting ready for discharge and is concerned that her older daughter may not accept the new baby. The nurse should suggest that:

a. the older daughter come to the hospital to take the baby home.
b. another adult play with the older child when the mother is caring for the baby.
c. the father carry the new baby and give the older child a doll.
d. Mrs. Hill give the older child more responsibility and assure her that she is now a big girl.

26-23
B
Appl.
Impl.

Mrs. Hill is concerned about when she and her husband can have sexual relations. The nurse should encourage the couple to wait until:

a. Mrs. Hill has had her 6-week check-up.
b. the episiotomy has healed and the lochia has stopped.
c. the lochia is no longer red and the vagina is nontender.
d. after the first menstrual period.

26-24
A
Comp.
Plan.

Mrs. Hill stated that after she had her last baby, intercourse was painful and she did not want it to be painful again. The nurse should explain that the pain resulted from:

a. decreased vaginal lubrication.
b. trauma to the vaginal mucosa.
c. increased maternal fatigue.
d. changes in the cervical os.

Cindy and Robert Andrus have delivered their first baby vaginally. Cindy is nursing the baby and the nurse is preparing the family for discharge.

(THE FOLLOWING 5 ITEMS RELATE TO THE ABOVE PASSAGE.)

26-25
C
Appl.
Impl.

When the nurse asked Cindy and Robert what type of birth control that they were planning to use, they stated that since Cindy is nursing they don't have to worry about birth control. The nurse should tell them that:

a. they can decide on a method when Cindy stops nursing.
b. no birth control is necessary until after the first menstrual period.
c. ovulation can occur when a woman is breast-feeding.
d. since Cindy has been pregnant once it will be much easier fo her to become pregnant now.

26-26
A
Appl.
Impl.

This is Cindy's third postpartum day. Cindy tells the nurse that she feels really sad and starts to cry easily. The nurse should explain that:

a. these feelings are normal and will decrease after the first week.
b. Cindy's physician will order an antidepressant for her to take at home.
c. If Cindy will focus on the fact that she has a healthy baby the feelings will decrease.
d. once Cindy is home with her family and friends she will not have these feelings.

26-27
D
Know.
Impl.

The nurse should prepare the couple for the fact that Cindy may have decreased sexual desire for:

a. 6 weeks.
b. 3 months.
c. 6 months.
d. 12 months.

151

26-28
A
Appl.
Impl.

After being home for 2 days, Cindy calls the nurse and states that she does not feel well and that her lochia is still bright red. The nurse should tell her to:

a. notify her physician about her symptoms.
b. decrease her activity and increase her fluid intake.
c. increase the frequency of the Kegel exercises.
d. take her temperature and call the doctor only if she has a fever.

26-29
C
Comp.
Plan.

Cindy is concerned that her baby cannot wait 4 hours between breast-feedings. The pediatrician's nurse explains to Cindy that she may need to adjust the baby's feeding schedule. The best adjustment at this time would be for every:

a. hour.
b. 1 to 2 hours.
c. 2 to 3 hours.
d. 3 to 4 hours.

Ginger Faraday has had a cesarean birth. She is a 24-year-old gravida 2. The nurse in the postpartal area checks Ginger frequently.

(THE FOLLOWING 3 ITEMS RELATE TO THE ABOVE PASSAGE.)

26-30
D
Comp.
Impl.

Which nursing action during the first day or two will improve intestinal motility?

a. Encourage leg exercises at least every 2 hours.
b. Help Ginger turn, cough, and deep breathe every 2 hours.
c. Provide frequent analgesics to minimize pain.
d. Have Ginger ambulate in her room.

26-31
D
Appl.
Impl.

The nurse wants to encourage Ginger to interact with her infant. Which of the following actions will facilitate this?

a. Provide environmental stimuli to improve Ginger's mental status.
b. Allow no visitors to interfere with Ginger and her infant.
c. Make decisions for Ginger so she can spend more time with her infant.
d. Focus Ginger's attention on the infant.

26-32
B
Comp.
Impl.

Ginger is experiencing some pains in her abdomen. After a nursing assessment of her complaint, the nurse finds Ginger may be experiencing gas pains. Which of the following nursing actions will assist in minimizing gas pains?

a. Avoid serving protein or solid foods for the first 48 hours.
b. Avoid giving Ginger a straw and carbonated drinks.
c. Give Ginger a hot drink several times a day.
d. Position Ginger in a semi-Fowler's position.

26-33
A
Appl.
Plan.

In order to provide an environment that is most conducive to bonding, the nurse should provide the Raines family with:

a. secure environment and time for the family to be together.
b. a home-like environment with all of the medical equipment hidden from view.
c. adequate time following birth for the mother to rest before having her care for the baby.
d. time for the mother and father to be alone together before interacting with the baby.

Noelle Zimmerman, 15 years old, has delivered her first baby vaginally.

(THE FOLLOWING 3 ITEMS RELATE TO THE ABOVE PASSAGE.)

26-34
B
Know.
Plan.

Because of Noelle's age, the nurse should encourage Noelle to have what kind of interaction with her baby?

a. visual
b. verbal
c. tactile
d. auditory

26-35
D
Appl.
Impl.

Which of the following examples of charting would objectively indicate that the mother has bonded to the infant?

a. Gave return bath demonstration.
b. Nursed the baby without difficulty.
c. Stated that she loves the baby.
d. Cuddled the baby and calls him by name.

26-36
A
Appl.
Impl.

Noelle tells the nurse that she is scared and doesn't know how to care for an infant. In order to help Noelle the nurse should:

a. be supportive and act as a role model.
b. discuss the possibility of adoption.
c. tell Noelle that her mother will help her.
d. tell Noelle that being a mother is an instinct.

26-37
B
Appl.
Impl.

The Kennedys have asked the nurse how they can help their 4-year-old daughter accept the new baby. The nurse should encourage them to:

a. have the older daughter share her bedroom with the infant.
b. include the older daughter in caring for the infant.
c. send the older daughter to a day-care center for half a day.
d. allow the older child to invite more friends over to play.

Chapter 27

The Postpartal Family at Risk

Instructions: For each of the following multiple-choice questions, select the ONE most appropriate answer.

Walter and Barbara Finnley have just delivered a 10-pound female. Midforceps were used and the estimated blood loss was 300 cc. Since birth, Barbara has had a large amount of lochia.

(THE FOLLOWING 5 ITEMS RELATE TO THE ABOVE PASSAGE.)

27-1
B
Comp.
Asses.

At birth the placenta and membrane are carefully inspected to determine:

a. which side of the placenta was expelled first.
b. if they were expelled intact.
c. the presence of vascular irregularities.
d. the number of veins and arteries.

27-2
C
Appl.
Diag.

Which of the following nursing diagnoses would have priority for Barbara?

a. possible retention of placental fragments
b. alteration in parenting skills
c. potential fluid volume deficit
d. alteration in comfort

27-3
D
Appl.
Impl.

During Barbara's assessment the nurse finds her lochia flow is heavy, and her uterus is boggy. The nurse should FIRST:

a. notify the obstetrician or midwife.
b. speed up the IV Pitocin.
c. help Barbara ambulate.
d. massage the fundus until it is firm.

27-4
C
Appl.
Impl.

Barbara's obstetrician performed bimanual uterine compression and the lochia has decreased. In order to provide safety for Barbara the nurse should:

a. massage the fundus every 15 minutes.
b. take the vital signs every 30 minutes.
c. check the lochia and uterine tone every 15 minutes.
d. have Barbara contract and relax the perineum every 30 minutes.

27-5
B
Appl.
Impl.

The care plan for Barbara states, "the nurse is to keep a pad count." In order for the nurse to carry out this intervention s/he should:

a. ask Barbara to count how many times she changes pads in a 24 hour period.
b. record the number of pads used and the amount of saturation.
c. record the percent of saturation of each pad after one hour of use.
d. record the number of pads used during her shift.

Carla Edwards has experienced an early postpartum hemorrhage. Her orders are: oxygen per face mask at 6 to 8 L/min., vital signs every 15 minutes, and IV Pitocin.

(THE FOLLOWING 3 ITEMS RELATE TO THE ABOVE PASSAGE.)

27-6
C
Appl.
Eval.

In order to assess whether the fluid volume replacement is adequate for Carla, the nurse should:

a. place Carla on daily weights.
b. assess her skin turgor for signs of dehydration.
c. assess the urinary output hourly.
d. regulate the IV to run at 125 cc/h.

27-7
A
Appl.
Impl.

Carla complains that she is really tired and has no energy. The nurse's best intervention would be to tell her:

a. the fatigue is a result of the blood loss.
b. she will slowly regain her energy in the next 2 weeks.
c. all postpartum clients are tired after labor and delivery.
d. she will feel better after a good night's sleep.

27-8
B
Appl.
Impl.

In order to promote bonding between Carla and her new baby, the nurse should:

a. encourage Carla to room-in with the infant.
b. bring the baby to Carla when she is comfortable.
c. have Carla feed the baby every 2 hours.
d. allow Carla to recover before having to cope with the infant.

Frank and Aletha Colby delivered their first baby vaginally with no problems. Aletha will be discharged from the hospital in 4 hours.

(THE FOLLOWING 3 ITEMS RELATE TO THE ABOVE PASSAGE.)

27-9
B
Appl.
Impl.

To prepare Aletha for discharge and to assure her adequate knowledge in the care of the newborn, the nurse's best instructions would concern:

a. the possibility of physiological jaundice in the newborn.
b. normal physiologic changes and how to assess them.
c. the signs and symptoms of colic.
d. the infant's prescribed feeding schedule.

27-10
D
Appl.
Impl.

The next day Aletha calls the postpartum unit and asks to speak to a nurse. She tells the nurse she has found a small lump or swelling on the perineum and doesn't know what to do about it. The nurse should tell Aletha to:

a. apply a warm compress to the area.
b. take a sitz bath twice a day.
c. elevate her hips and legs as much as possible.
d. apply an ice pack to the area.

27-11   To relieve associated discomfort, the nurse should suggest that Aletha:
A
Appl.   a. take an analgesic.
Impl.   b. do Kendal exercises.
         c. gently puncture the swelling with a sterile needle.
         d. decrease her activity and elevate her hips and legs.

Lisa Redmond, 15 years old, has delivered her first child.

(THE FOLLOWING 3 ITEMS RELATE TO THE ABOVE PASSAGE.)

27-12   The vagina and uterus of most women at the time of birth:
C
Know.   a. are sterile.
Asses.   b. contain no pathogens.
         c. have pathogenic organisms that are capable of causing infection.
         d. are infected if the membranes have been ruptured more than 24 hours.

27-13   The nurse carefully explains perineal care to Lisa. Lisa's understanding and
A   and follow-through of perineal care is important primarily to:
Know.
Impl.   a. decrease the possibility of infection.
         b. increase Lisa's comfort.
         c. speed healing of the perineum.
         d. help shrink the hemorrhoids.

27-14   Which of the following occurrences would alert the nurse to the fact that Lisa
C   is at risk for postpartum infection?
Comp.
Analy.   a. delivery of a 6-pound baby
         b. vaginal delivery after 1 hour of pushing
         c. prenatal malnutrition
         d. rupture of membranes 2 hours before birth

Rich and Ginger James have delivered their third baby by cesarean birth. Ginger
plans to breast-feed the baby and have the infant room-in.

(THE FOLLOWING 6 ITEMS RELATE TO THE ABOVE PASSAGE.)

27-15   It is Ginger's first day postpartum. How often should her temperature be taken?
C
Appl.   a. q 2 h.
Plan.   b. t.i.d.
         c. q.i.d.
         d. b.i.d.

27-16   When the nurse changes the bandages on Ginger's incision, s/he observes the skin
B   edges of the incision are red, edematous, and tender to touch. The nurse's best
Appl.   intervention would be to:
Impl.
         a. cleanse the wound with hydrogen peroxide.
         b. chart her observations and notify the obstetrician.
         c. chart her observation of the first phase of the normal healing process.
         d. observe the incision closely for the next 24 to 48 hours.

27-17
C
Appl.
Impl.

The nurse's assessment of Ginger reveals an elevation in her temperature, chills, nausea, and increased pain. The nurse notifies the primary physician and receives the following orders: ampicillin in 500 mg IV q 6 h, culture and sensitivity of lochia, ultrasound of the pelvis, and chest x-ray. Which order should the nurse carry out first?

a. ultrasound.
b. IV antibiotic
c. culture of lochia
d. chest x-ray

27-18
C
Appl.
Impl.

The physician removes Ginger's sutures from her abdominal incision and the wound gapes open. Ginger asks the nurse, "Why did the doctor remove my stitches? Obviously I am not healed yet." The nurse's best reply would be:

a. "The stitches had to be removed because they were infected."
b. "Your doctor will replace the stitches with stronger, hypoallergenic ones."
c. "Removing the stitches will allow the infected incision to drain."
d. "This will allow the incision to heal from the inside out."

27-19
A
Appl.
Impl.

Ginger has been placed on isolation and the baby can no longer room-in. In order to promote bonding between the mother and infant, the nurse should:

a. provide a picture of the baby for Ginger.
b. have the father visit the baby more often.
c. assure Ginger she will be in isolation only a short time.
d. encourage Ginger to spend the time away from the baby resting so she will recover faster.

27-20
B
Comp.
Analy.

Since Ginger cannot breast-feed her baby while she is in isolation, she must pump her breasts. The MOST important reason for Ginger to pump her breasts is to:

a. prevent engorgement.
b. assure continued milk production.
c. remove the infected milk.
d. promote uterine involution.

Bud and Nancy Cox have delivered their first baby by cesarean birth.

(THE FOLLOWING 5 ITEMS RELATE TO THE ABOVE PASSAGE.)

27-21
B
Know.
Asses.

Which of the following maternal factors would predispose Nancy to thrombophlebitis?

a. early ambulation
b. maternal obesity
c. use of a nonestrogen lactation suppressant
d. increased intake of calcium-rich foods

157

27-22
B
Know.
Asses

The symptoms of thrombophlebitis will usually appear on the _____ postpartum day.

a. first
b. third
c. seventh
d. tenth

27-23
A
Comp.
Impl.

To prevent thrombophlebitis, the nurse should:

a. encourage early ambulation.
b. provide increased fluids to enhance circulation.
c. massage Nancy's legs b.i.d.
d. impose strict bed rest for the first 72 hours postpartum.

27-24
A
Comp.
Diag.

The nurse believes Nancy may have a pulmonary emboli. Which of the following assessment data would lead the nurse to this conclusion?

a. sudden dyspnea, sweating, confusion, and hypotension
b hypertension, hemoptysis, cyanosis, and coughing
c. chest pain, hemoptysis, and hypertension
d. chills, fever, pain, and syncope

27-25
D
Comp.
Impl.

Nancy will be discharged on warfarin. Discharge teaching should include which of the following safety instructions regarding this medication? The nurse should tell Dorothy to:

a. avoid walking long distances and climbing stairs.
b. avoid any lacerations, punctures, or bruising type injuries.
c. keep an injectable form of warfarin available.
d. avoid taking aspirin and certain anti-inflammatory drugs.

Albert and Dorothy Hamilton delivered an 8-pound baby girl 30 minutes ago.

(THE FOLLOWING 3 ITEMS RELATE TO THE ABOVE PASSAGE.)

27-26
C
Comp.
Asses.

During Dorothy's initial postpartal assessment, the nurse will assess the bladder. Which of the following observations would indicate an over-distended bladder?

a. positive Homans' sign
b. voiding measured at 200 cc
c. lower pelvic mass
d. Dorothy's complaint of discomfort while voiding

27-27
C
Appl.
Impl.

Dorothy is to undergo catheterization. As the nurse explains the procedure, Dorothy asks if the procedure is painful. The nurse's best response would be:

a. "Catheterization is painless."
b. "You will feel pressure but no pain."
c. "The procedure may be uncomfortable but relaxation will help."
d. "You will feel a burning sensation as the tube enters your bladder."

27-28   The nurse inserts the catheter and removes 1000 cc of urine from Dorothy's bladder.
B   What should s/he do at this time?
Appl.
Impl.
     a. Remove the catheter and encourage Dorothy to void any remaining urine in the bladder.
     b. Clamp the catheter for 1 hour.
     c. Continue to drain urine from the bladder until the bladder is empty.
     d. Remove the catheter and instruct Dorothy in Kegel exercises to strengthen the contractions of the bladder.

George and Kathy Wood delivered their third child 2 days ago.

(THE FOLLOWING 2 ITEMS RELATE TO THE ABOVE PASSAGE.)

27-29   In order to determine if Kathy is at risk for psychological maladjustment, the nurse
D   should ask Kathy:
Appl.
Impl.
     a. her age at the time her first baby was born.
     b. if she feels confident in caring for the baby.
     c. about the family income and fixed expenses.
     d. how she reacted to the birth of her other children.

27-30   Kathy is diagnosed as suffering from depression. Prior to discharge the nurse
A   should:
Comp.
Plan.
     a. refer Kathy to a public health nurse.
     b. arrange for short-term hospitalization in a private psychiatric facility.
     c. develop an exercise program for her so she cannot sit around and become further depressed.
     d. notify the community children's protective services and have them evaluate the home environment.

NOTES

NOTES

NOTES

NOTES

NOTES

NOTES

NOTES

NOTES

NOTES